I0454781

War Against Cancer
Cancer Control: Holistic Approach, 312 Pages

Dr. Arvind Kulkarni, a well-known radiation oncologist and researcher in alternative medicine, has done a wonderful job of providing new insights into causation, prevention and holistic treatment strategies for cancer. *War Against Cancer,* written primarily forlay public, provides useful information in simple terms, about various ways to successfully fight cancer. The book covers all the aspects of the big "C".

Post September 11th, the world has changed. We all have become acutely aware of the need to fight terrorism at every step. Cancer is the internal terrorism, rebellion by some of our own body cells. The bad news is that by violating natural laws of the health, we might be responsible for the risk. The good news is that with re-orientation of our mental attitudes, nutrition and lifestyles, we might overcome this enemy.

There are many similarities between origin, promotion and spread of cancer affecting the body and the terrorist menace affecting the world. In addition to prevalent methods of surgery, radiation and chemotherapy, we need a long-term strategy to address the root causes of cancer; why and how it started in the first place. We have to take care of the soil (body) as well as the seed (cancer cells). The book should prove very useful to cancer patients, their relatives and friends and to anyone who desires to learn more about cancer problem.

War Against Cancer
By
Arvind V. Kulkarni, M.D.

COPY RIGHT
Mrs. Shreelekha Kulkarni
H-52 Dalamal Park
223 Cuffe Parade
Mumbai 400005
India

Phone: (91-20) -67346000
Email: kulkarni_arvind@hotmail.com

Hard Copy First Published in India 2003
Reprint 2008

www.ayurved-for-cancer.org

**Integrated Cancer Treatment & Research Center,
Wagholi, Pune 412207, MS, INDIA**

ictrcpune@gmail.com

Dedicated to the memory of my mother

Dr. Laxmibai Kulkarni

*Ideal Mother
And A Bright Ayurvedic Physician
Who bravely fought her
War Against Cancer
till the end*

CONTENTS

Preface

Foreword

ABOUT THE AUTHOR

Dr Arvind V. Kulkarni, a well-known cancer specialist, graduated in Medicine from the B.J.Medical College, Pune in 1963. He did his post-graduate specialization abroad, securing a Diploma in Radiology from the Liverpool University and a Fellowship in Radiation Oncology from the New York University. After practising in New York, Dr. Kulkarni returned to Mumbai in 1973. Initially he worked at the Jaslok Hospital and later at the Bombay Hospital as Head of Radiation Oncology Department.

A few years into his profession, Dr Kulkarni realized the limitations of Surgery, Radiation and Chemotherapy, therapeutic procedures available to fight cancer, but which did not address the underlying causes. Further, administration of Radiation and Chemotherapy deprived the body of its natural defences significantly making it weak and susceptible to other infections.

Intent on enhancing the quality of this conventional care, Dr. Kulkarni turned to complementary alternative therapies like Ayurveda and Homeopathy. He initiated in 1985, clinical research trials along with a few colleagues having a similar bent of mind. The composite therapy thus evolved could bring immense relief to patients undergoing Radiation and Chemotherapy, by controlling the side effects and pain, normally associated with such curative techniques.

In 1998, Allegheny University Hospital in Pittsburgh, USA invited Dr. Kulkarni to work as the Director of Integrated Medicine. Around the same time, the American College of Advancement in Medicine, an institution engaged in pioneering research work in complementary Alternative Medicine also awarded its membership to him. Dr. Kulkarni is a Diplomat of the American Board of Radiology.

PREFACE

For 35 years, I have been a Radiation Oncologist serving more than 15000 patients in India, the UK and USA. Like any beginner, I too believed that pills, machines and incisions could cure all diseases. I had great pride in Radiotherapy techniques and the 'cure' it brought about in many of my patients. Failures after all were a part of the medical statistics!

As years went by, I started realising that the triad of Surgery, Radiation and Chemotherapy needed support to improve the quality of life of a cancer patient. Chasing a tumour or its shadow in an X-ray was insufficient. Any treatment, irrespective of its nature had to focus simultaneously on the disease as well as the patient. It was similar to nurturing both the soil and seeds with equal attention to derive a better yield. In 1973 while at the Jaslok Hospital, I had to perform a radium implantation operation on a patient suffering from third stage cancer of the uterus. Seeing her condition, Vaidya S. S. Bhave, a colleague of mine hesitatingly asked me if he could try out Ayurvedic medications on her. Since there was hardly anything further to do, I gave him the green signal. Under Vaidya Bhave's care, supplementing the main course of radiation treatments, the patient started showing rapid improvement. She had fewer side reactions. Later on, in the periodic check-ups, she appeared a picture of health and for almost 25 years thereafter was free of the disease. .

This incident prompted me to turn to Vaidya Bhave for more inputs on Ayurveda. He found my unprejudiced approach encouraging and happily acquainted me with *Sushrut Samhita*, the famed Ayurvedic text. Its complex narration or basic tenets of application did not intimidate me. Perhaps, genetically I had an affinity for this ancient medical science. My mother Dr. Laxmibai Kulkarni was a well-known Ayurvedic physician. She died of cancer fighting it bravely until the end. My mother's competence and confidence in Ayurveda must have left a deep impact on me. I never realised it then or until a few years after my return on completion of the training abroad in oncology.

Around this time, I happened to meet Vaidya Sadanand Sardeshmukh in Mumbai. His intuitive healing powers and mastery over Ayurveda were amazing. We joined hands to research the effects of Ayurveda on cancer patients. Poojya Sardeshmukh Maharaj, father of Vaidya Sardeshmukh impressed with our work, suggested that we set up a Cancer Research Project at their Ayurvedic Research Centre in Pune. I am glad that this project initiated in 1994 is progressing as envisaged. Vaidya Narendra Pendse whom I came across in the early 1990s was another bright young Ayurvedic consultant from Pune to collaborate with me in such studies.

Leading Homeopathic practitioners such as Dr.Gunavante, Dr Rajan Sankaran, Dr. Jawahar Shah and others impressed me so much that I even attended a special course in Homeopathy. Dr Lara Shah, an established Homeopath helped me in my efforts to formulate a treatment mode for cancer patients. While, we found Homeopathy effective in controlling the sufferings and side reactions of modern cancer therapies, it did not offer a ready cure for cancer. Many Homeopaths, I know, would differ with me on this subject. I also experimented with Acupuncture, Meditation and even Hypnotherapy.

In 1998, Allegheny General Hospital at Pittsburgh in the USA invited me to work as the Medical Director of Integrated Medicine. A wave of Complementary Medicine was then sweeping all over America, Europe and other developed countries. Dr. Paul Lebovitz and Ms. Kathleen Krebs of the Integrated Medicine Department helped me get a wide exposure in this field. Trailblazers like Dr. James Gordon of Georgetown University, Dr Herbert Benson from Harvard, Dr. Bernie Siegel from New Haven and Dr. Andrew Weils from Arizona, also motivated me a great deal.

Modern Medicine by virtue of its established procedures and accomplishments over the last many decades enjoys an unparalleled position. When it fails to ensure a cure or induces side reactions, we tend to seek support and solace from other treatment methods commonly referred to as 'Alternative Medicine'. My endeavour has been to devise a holistic approach in the treatment of cancer. In this, I have been fortunate to receive unqualified guidance and co-operation from the right people at the right time. I believe efforts of these and other open-minded scientists all over the world would give a new direction and impetus to the 21st century medicine.

The environment at the Bombay Hospital with which I was associated for a long time also turned out to be conducive to my experiments in composite therapy. Professional colleagues however chose to view my efforts with circumspection. Some of them branded me a 'quack' doctor, while the silent majority expressed a passing interest in the matter.

'War Against Cancer' reflects all that I could experience, observe and learn during all these years. For quite sometime, I have been toying with the idea of sharing this with the outer world. If it has materialised now, the entire credit must go to my wife Shreelekha. She has been a source of inspiration and support. She constantly egged me on to complete the manuscript as early as possible, reading it carefully and offering her criticisms and suggestions. I am also grateful to my friend Mr D. R. Nayar for his painstaking effort in going through the manuscript and offering valuable suggestions in its final presentation.

I must caution that the opinions expressed here are purely personal. It may or may not find ready acceptance with all. Further, I have neither suggested nor implied any claim or assurance in the name of a cure for cancer. Cancer is a serious disease. Whatever be the line of treatment, it needs the direct supervision and care of a competent medical practitioner. Doctors can only treat; the cure has to come from within you. Remember the old adage "Doctors treat; He heals".

CHAPTER 1

WAR AGAINST CANCER!

SEPTEMBER 11th:
In the beginning of the 21st Century and especially after September 11th it would be necessary to take a second look at our approach to Cancer Problem. Cancer problem can very well be compared to "Terrorist Problem". Terrorist problem affects the whole world while the Cancer Problem affects the whole body. Both the problems are in the making for several years before the actual explosive diagnosis. Both the problems have tremendous physical, psychological as well as spiritual implications.

The *Vedas* (ancient Hindu Scriptures) state that human body is miniature world! *"Whatever is in pinda, the same is in brahmanda"*! A *dosha (*disturbances) in one part of the world eventually affect the whole world. Persistent *dosha* in one part of the body, if not corrected, can eventually affect the whole body. In the outer world as well as within the body, disturbances can manifest either as acute or chronic problems in different parts.

Terrorist mentality was in the making over the past many years. The world community, preoccupied with its own welfare, usually ignored the remote disturbances. A local problem was thought to be an insignificant symptom, which would somehow go away. When the World Trade Center in New York crumpled, it was then a confirmed diagnosis of terrorist cancer affecting the whole world.

Human body has more than 50 billion cells. Carcinogens are external chemical, physical and biological influences, which are known to promote cancer. Under the influences of persistent unhealthy life styles and exposures to carcinogens, some groups of body cells start their "malignant"covert activities. If the soil is ready, the disturbance takes root and a visible cancer tumor is soon noticed.

Why Cancer?

Unhealthy life styles and exposures to cancer causing chemicals are important, but not the exclusive causes of cancer. There are many other known and unknown factors initiating the cancer process. Cancer is sometimes seen in very young children who obviously could not have had any bad habits. On the other hand, we see many people full of so called bad habits apparently enjoying good health. This compels us to consider some other factors in childhood cancer. Pregnant mothers, who are exposed to carcinogens, may be transmitting such influences to the fetus in the womb. A baby might be born with susceptibility to cancer. This susceptibility may be genetic in origin. Hindu philosophy has concept of repeated cycles of birth and death. *Vedas* stress consequences of *karma*, good and bad deeds performed in this and earlier life. As you sow, so shall you reap. Could these karma in the past lives manifest through genes in this life bringing us to various good or bad experiences?

There are special genes called oncogenes in our body cells. Protective Oncogenes can resist cancer. However, when "turned on" or "altered" the same genes could promote cancer. What turns these oncogenes "on"? What causes a cell either to fight cancer or to join cancer? Carcinogens are outside substances, which can trigger oncogenes and develop cancer. Carcinogens are external things such as tobacco, pollution, pesticides, chemicals, drugs, radiation, x-rays, ultra-violet rays, old or chronic injuries to the body, chronic infections etc. The internal factors are host factors. A person may be born with genetic susceptibility to develop a cancer more easily than others. Such susceptible persons, if exposed to carcinogens, can easily develop cancer. On the other hand, if such persons carefully avoid exposure to carcinogens, they can reduce the risk of getting cancer. Recent medical research suggests that under the persistent influence of carcinogens, oncogenes can become activated and start cancer. It has been shown in the research laboratories that persistent exposure to carcinogens can reduce immunity, which is the natural disease fighting power. With reduced immunity, various diseases can take hold of the body. Mental depression and anxiety can reduce immunity. Fortunately it has been also proved in laboratories that good healthy natural food, exercise, regular habits, relaxation, meditation, yoga, cheerful attitude and even good sleep can improve immunity. Such measures would help one to fight many diseases.

Focus of Allopathy:
Allopathic medicine usually considers only physical aspects of a disease. With few exceptions, allopathy treats diseases on a physical level alone. Although we all are aware of the existence of mind and spirit behind the body, these entities cannot be shown in the test tubes. These subtle realities are discounted when an allopathic doctor treats physical diseases such as infection, diabetes, blood pressure, cancer etc. Allopathic medicine is like a fire fighter. When there is an actual fire, the fire brigade will rush and extinguish the fire quickly by whatever means available. However, fire prevention is more important in the long run.

When body develops an acute disease, a medical doctor will prescribe the required antibiotic, anti-fever, anti-diarrhea, anti-acid, anti-pain, anti-sleep, anti-bleeding, anti-tension, anti-convulsion, anti-cancer pills etc. No doubt this quick fixing medicine works wonders and immediately arrests the symptoms of a disease. However, we should remember that human body is a miraculous machine, which is usually able to heal itself. Many of the symptoms such as fever, diarrhea, cough, sweating, pain etc could reflect natural healing process. Undue interference with such processes might lead to other chronic health problems in the long run. In modern age, in spite of more hospitals, more doctors, more drugs and more advances, there seem to be more ill health. Modern medicine is becoming more and more mechanical, complicated and less affordable for an average individual. Modern medicine has no satisfactory answers to many chronic diseases. Indulgence in bad habits, unhealthy food, impure water, polluted air, and mental stresses may be responsible for ill health on large scale.

That is why Alternative Medicine is getting more and more popular all over the world.

Alternative Medicine:
Alternative medicine is not one specific medical science. It is a basket of different systems prevalent in various parts of the world. Most of these systems are time tested old methods. Some are new and are being explored. The common approach of these methods is to attend to the whole body, including mind. Treat the body and mind together. Empower your own mind and body to fight your own disease. That is the common basis for various alternative medical systems. These methods not only treat the symptoms or laboratory findings of a disease but also try to go at the root cause of the disease. These systems emphasize disease prevention. Modern medicine has made lot of important advances and some of these are life saving in acute medical condition and accidents. Alternative medicine many times tries to complement modern medicine. Hence, alternative medicine is also known by other names such as Complementary Alternative Medicine, Integrated Medicine, and Holistic Medicine. Ayurved figures prominently in the list of alternative medical sciences.

There is worldwide interest in Ayurveda and other alternative medical sciences. National Institutes of Health in USA has recently established a special division called National Center for Complementary and Alternative Medicine in Washington, DC. This center promotes research in various alternative medical systems. The center has published a list of various alternative medical sciences prevalent in different parts of the world. The list includes Ayurveda, Yoga, Meditation, Homeopathy, Energy Medicine, Mind-Body Medicine, Acupuncture, Chinese Medicine, Herbal Medicine, Naturopathy, Nutritional Medicine, Reiki and many more. National Cancer Institute, another branch of NIH, has a special section to do research on cancer treatment with alternative medicine. There is keen interest in Ayurveda all over the world. In a latest study by Dr. Eisenberg, published in the Journal of American Medical Association in 1998, it was shown that almost 40 % of all the Americans take some help from Alternative

Medical Practitioners every year. The same is true in other parts of the world.

We are fortunate to have Ayurveda as our heritage. However, we have to do medical research with modern methods to study Ayurveda and learn the exact scope of Ayurveda in various chronic diseases. We should not be prejudiced, either for or against Ayurveda. Research based evidence can guide us about proper scope of Ayurveda. Ayurveda is not a dead science but it is a dynamic science. We could take help of other medical sciences, if needed, to understand ayurveda better. Whatever is written in old textbooks should be verified for our own understanding. Blind faith is as dangerous as blind logic. Later on in this book, detailed information is given about the Cancer Research Project being conducted at Ayurved Hospital and Research center at Wagholi, Pune.

War Against Cancer:
War Against Cancer is similar to the War Against Terrorism. Terrorists are the members of the society who have taken a wrong turn. Cancer cells are formed from our own cells, which have gone out of control. They serve no useful purpose but attack other peace loving hard working parts of our body. Like terrorists, cancer cells can spread from one area to another, causing pain and suffering. Terrorists may hide within civilian population. Cancer tumor is present within body surrounded by normal cells. Bombardment of terrorist camps may destroy some terrorist if you can get them precisely. Some collateral civilian damage is unavoidable. Similarly, with chemotherapy and radiation, some damage to surrounding normal organs is unavoidable. After destruction of cancer, re-building of body is more important. Ayurveda and other Alternative Medical Sciences can enable your own body to prevent cancer cells from conducting terrorist activity. Individual terrorists can be killed but as long as terror mentality persists in the society, more terrorists will come. Similarly, we can destroy cancer tumor, but as long as the basic disturbances are not corrected, cancer can come back. Rehabilitation of body and empowerment of immunity is critical for eradication of cancer.

The aim of this book is to make reader aware of the nature of cancer problem and provide information about various treatment strategies to deal with cancer. In subsequent chapters, I will try to express my personal views about causes, diagnosis and treatment of cancer. True stories of some unusual cancer patients will be given. Role of mind in causation as well as control of cancer will be highlighted. Some complementary cancer therapies will be briefly described. "Check-list for Action" and "Diet Instructions to Fight Cancer" will be included in the appendix at the end. Success of each strategy may vary greatly from patient to patient. There may not be any guarantee of cure with any of these methods. The advice given in this book is for general information only. If you have a specific health problem, you should take help of a competent medical professional in the treatment of your disease. You should be the soldier in your war against cancer, but you still need a competent commanding officer to call the shots in your War Against Cancer.

CHAPTER 2

HEALTH SCENARIO, Past, Present & Future

Where are we today, in health matters, as we stand in the door of the new century, new millennium? We have come far ahead of our stone age, middle age and also ahead of our industrial age, which was progressing for the past 300 years or so. We are now in computer age, Internet age, and communication age.

Only 100 years ago, common man could not have dreamt of Space Shuttles, Man on Moon, Instant conversation across the globe, email, the World Wide Web, and video pictures by Internet. Computers, space travel, landing on other planets, internet information web, map of human genome and many other discoveries enriched material life for the whole humanity beyond imagination. A man in one part of the world can become suddenly aware of the NEWS in other parts the world, thanks to the TV and Internet technology. Information spreads fast, like a wild fire. We are bombarded with information every second. This we call knowledge. Knowledge is that which gives us happiness, satisfaction. As stated by Lord Gautam Buddha," Knowledge is that, which Liberates!" Are we more satisfied, happier than, say, than our parents or the generations before? As a famous poet said before, " Where is the knowledge in this endless information and where is the wisdom in this endless knowledge?" What is the difference between information, knowledge and wisdom?

What is the aim of human life? Are we on this planet only for the material enjoyment? Are we here only for recreation and procreation and to amass material wealth? The reality, which dawns at different times for different persons, tells us otherwise. No matter how much successful we are in the outer world, it is our inner world which counts. Happiness, satisfaction, love, sense of fulfillment comes from within. This is not to say that the outer achievements are illusory, not worth pursuing. If the humanity has to progress to higher goals, we need a balance between the progress outside and the progress within, The 20th Century was for the exploration of the outer world. The 21st Century would be for exploration of the inner world that is our mind, our spirit. Unless we seek this, there will be no real happiness, health and peace for humanity.

Human Body: A Miracle Machine:
The art of medicine was born with the birth of first man. It had to be. Human body was subjected to the strife, internal as well as external, right from the beginning. "Avoid pain" must have been one of the earliest preoccupations of the mankind. All the nature is subject to continuous modifications. Nothing stands still. Even stones on the mountains get disintegrated slowly over the millennia. The cycles of creation, sustenance and then destruction go on as per the nature's clock.

Human body is a miracle of the nature. If you believe in God, you can call it a gift from God. Creation of human body was not a random accident of the nature. It is the work of cosmic intelligence, a divine plan, for a definite higher purpose. Body is a self maintaining, regulating, correcting wonder machine of the nature. The pump, called heart, beats day and night, without gap, for the whole life! The computer, called the brain, thinks and organizes all the activities, day and night, even during sleep. It does not depend on any external electrical supply, which is liable for interruption. Similarly, all the organs; liver, lungs, kidneys, intestines etc do their job day and night without any demands for wage hikes or benefits.

Only when some of our organs are abused due to our own folly, the disease gets a foothold. Violation of natural laws of health is responsible for more than 90 % of the diseases. These problems are usually preventable or could be kept under reasonable control. However, each person is born with specific genetic disposition. This variety can create a variety of health problems, without any apparent reasons, at any age. Even if a person is genetically prone to get certain disease, it might be possible to delay the onset of that disease or to slow down its progress, if proper steps are taken in time.

Medicine in Ancient Times:
Let us now review the status of health and medical science in the past and in the present. The available descriptions of medical practices date back more than 5000 years. Longevity, a measure of good health, was low in the past allover the world. In India, at the time of the independence, average longevity was said to be around 18- 20 years. Most of the people used to die of acute infections, epidemics. Infants and children died of malnutrition, infections. Those who survived usually lived long without much of chronic health problems. Wars, accidents, epidemics, infections and starving were common causes of death.

Various medical systems were evolved locally in different parts of the world to relieve suffering and disease. Ayurved in India and Chinese Medicine in China have texts dating back to 3000 to 4000 years. In the west, Egyptians were among the first to use some herbs. Methods for dealing with fractures and accidental wounds have been mentioned in all the ancient systems of medicine. Surgery was practiced in India, Egypt and China.

Greeks added their concepts of four humors to the Egyptian and Babylonian systems of medicine. These 4 humors were said to be blood, black bile, yellow bile and phlegm, which needed be in good balance for optimal health. Hippocrates, known as the father of western medicine was the outstanding physician of ancient Greece. Various superstitions of that time were slowly corrected. After the breakup of the Roman Empire, the tradition of the Egyptian medicine continued in various Arabian schools.

In parallel, Ayurved evolved the concepts of *Dosha, Dhatu and Mala.* In Ayurved, Dosha refers to three basic constituent principles of body, i.e. kapha, pitta and vata. Dhatus are seven tissue systems and Mala are the excretions from the body. This subject will be elaborated in later chapters. The concept of the creation of the universe with Panch-Mahabhoota, i.e. space, air, fire, water and earth, originated with Hindu rishis. Similar concepts of 5 elements creating the universe originated in China. Even in Christian Bible, there is a mention of the Word leading to formation of air, fire and water to create the earth. Local physicians trained in the local systems of the medicines were treating people. We do not have any statistical records of utility or the benefits of these systems at that time. However we have reason to believe that chronic diseases were much less common in earlier times, in spite of high mortality due to wars, infections and epidemics.

Industrial Age Medicine:
After the 17th century, Europeans began to seek a scientific basis for medical knowledge instead of relying on old Greek and Arabian texts. Many principles of anatomy and physiology were discovered by western scientist from 17th century onwards and the process still continues. The art of surgery was developed in 17th century England. The advent of chloroform and ether revolutionized surgical techniques. Various drugs were extracted from herbs, which were earlier used for treatment. Digitalis, Vitamin C, Aspirin are only few examples of the beginning of drug industry in the West.

In the East, physicians were content with old time tested formulations for treating diseases. In the East, physicians in India and China were studying the effects of the whole herbs. They could not and did not chemically analyze each herb in search of the active principle. Perhaps, they thought that proof of pudding was in eating! With European Industrial Revolution, the sciences of chemistry, physics, pathology, microbiology, mechanics, electricity, mathematics, statistics etc made rapid advances. This was due to analytical, enquiring western mind. The entire phenomenon needed the scientific proof to be believed. The theory of germs causing diseases was established. Smallpox vaccine was announced as the breakthrough experiment in immunization by Edward Jenner in 1798. John Morgan in Philadelphia established first medical school in America in 1765.

At about same time, Samuel Hahnemann in Germany discovered the science of homeopathy. An allopathic doctor disillusioned with the then prevalent medical practices, Hahnemann experimented on himself and his friends for his discovery of homeopathy. This was simply a bright scientific discovery to deal with diseases. Homeopathy became popular in Europe and America in 19th century and early 20th century. However with the onslaught of modern drug industry in the west, homeopathy soon fell back as an unproven medical science. In the changing worldwide health scenario over the past few decades, alternative medical sciences including homeopathy are now again coming back in prominence.

Medical Discoveries:
There is a series of brilliant medical discoveries in the last couple of centuries. In 1857, Louise Pasteur refined the germ theory of disease. In 1876, Robert Koch discovered the bacteria associated with tuberculosis and laid the foundation for bacteriology. In 1895, Wilhelm Roentgen in Germany discovered X rays, which revolutionized the medical diagnosis and treatment. Soon in 1898, Madam Curie discovered radium, laying foundation for the science of radioactivity and nuclear physics. In 1921, Banting and Best jointly isolated insulin, which revolutionized treatment of diabetes. Alexander Fleming in 1928 discovered penicillin, starting the era of antibiotics. All these discoveries gave great promises to cure all the diseases. However, after years of usage of the modern pharmaceuticals, their merits as well as demerits, shortcomings, limitations and drawbacks have now come under closer scrutiny.

The Second World War gave further impetus to scientific discoveries. In medical field, more diagnostic tools such as CT scan, MRI scan, Nuclear Scan, Ultrasound Scan and a number of other techniques were developed to monitor internal organs and their functions. Surgical techniques were further refined. The age of transplant was ushered. Kidney transplant, liver transplant, muscle transplant, joint replacement became household words. Man thought that nothing is impossible. With his science, man thought he could conquer the nature and overcome the disease, once and for all.

Pharmaceutical Industry:
The modern pharmaceutical industry embarked upon the search of the so-called active principle for every drug. Initially appealing to human logic and scientific tenets, various components were isolated from the plants known to have some medicinal value. Man wanted to do better than the nature. Hoping to refine a medicinal herb, it was subjected to incessant laboratory analysis, animal experiment and standardization. The end result was claimed to be a magic pill, with known action and known dose to produce a certain effect. This was good for the progress of medicine as well as for the progress of the industry. An herb costing pennies could be converted and sold as expensive pills or injections. The cost of medicines went up. All these research was directed to finding a specific action on the tissue. It was a quick fixing solution for a single bio-chemical anomaly assumed to be responsible for a specific disease. It was forgotten that disease process is much more complicated that works on multiple levels in the Mind-Body complex, which we call a Human. This was against the holistic approach to health.

Herbal Medicines:
A whole herb may have multiple synergistic components acting in unison to produce certain effects. The totality of action of an herb may be beyond our current scientific analysis. Our current scientific means may be unable to understand holistic pharmacology of actions of various natural products on the living humans. Man has mind and body. Animal experiments with single active principle may not accurately forecast effects of an herb on human body and mind. When you see a beautiful woman, you do not go in search of the active principle in that person to find what really turns you on! You do not analyze whether it is the eyes, or the hair, or the skin color or the lips, which is turning you on. If you isolate each of these parts, the effects will be not the same as the whole. It is the whole that is having composite action on the observer. Further, the action may vary also with the observer.

With the progress of the drug industry, there are now many synthetic drugs, which try to mimic the theoretical molecular structure of the original natural substance. Science is constantly evolving. Many scientific truths of the past centuries could not withstand the scrutiny of the current methods. The earth is now found to be round and revolving around the sun. In the European middle ages, earth was thought to be flat and the sun revolving round the earth. Such were the scientific beliefs of middle ages! One should keep the mind open in case our current scientific beliefs get challenged in the future. The theories of elements, molecules and atoms have undergone a sea change in the past 50 years. Atom was considered to be the smallest indivisible unit of mass. Einstein's new understanding of the physics is now modifying Newton's rigid laws of gravity, mass and energy. The current mechanistic pharmaceutical research does not address the holistic nature of human health and disease. This is the drawback of the modern drug discoveries.

Cost of Progress:
It is now obvious that the industrial revolution has offered us the prosperity and pleasure at the cost of pollution, inflation, ecological ruin, social unrest, isolation and mental stress. For commercial benefits, forests are being chopped, rivers polluted, toxic fumes released into air. Although man lives longer, he does not know inner peace and happiness. Human body has become storehouse of toxic wastes from the environment, food, water, air and also from indiscriminate use of modern drugs. A body, which has got terrorists hidden within, cannot function efficiently. It will complain. It will have variety of physical and mental problems. This translates into chronic health problems, which never seem to get cured. High blood pressure, diabetes, heart attack, cancer, arthritis, bowel disease, ulcers, depression, anxiety, fatigue, restlessness, loss of sleep, loss of appetite, bad moods etc seem to have become the order of the day. No doubt, many of these diseases might have some genetic predisposition. However, genes are also subject to mutations due to exposure to abnormal external and internal conditions.

Man and the World:
There are similarities in causes of social disturbances and causes of a disease. In a social violence, there is a long-standing discontent in some social groups due to the lack of corrective steps. There is failure of the detective intelligence to foresee any potential social disasters. Timely precautions and intervention could prevent the social disasters, or at least minimize their impact. Similarly, human body, if subjected to neglect and chronic abuse, can revolt and lead to a rebellion we call a disease. After all, human body is a miniature universe. Whatever is in Brahmanda, it is within Pinda! Microcosm is a miniature of macrocosm. Human body functions in a same way as a society functions. The society has countless groups of people to do specialized functions. Human body has countless individual cells and some organs for special functions. In health, each organ and all the cells work in a complementary fashion. The welfare of the whole body is the aim. Organs do not complain against each other. There are no strikes, lockouts, gherao or bandha! The health is disturbed only when there is an imbalance.

Current Health Scenario:
With more medical discoveries, more doctors and more hospitals, there seem to be more ill health, more dissatisfaction, and more unrest in the society. Although life expectancy has significantly increased, so have the chronic medical problems. Most of the chronic problems like high blood pressure, diabetes, arthritis, heart disease, cancer etc cannot be cured but can be kept under control. A person has to live and perhaps die with these conditions. Doctors can only make the life of such patients more tolerable, less painful. If by some miracle the condition does not go away, such persons have to be on medicines life long.

There must be some basic cause for this massive ill health affecting millions across the world. Medical advances, which have provided us with wonderful quick fixing pills, may not be adequate to offer us long-term health. The cure of our health problems, which are usually the results of our own violations of the Nature's Laws, has to come from within. The disease affects us on physical, mental and spiritual levels.

That is why we have to fight the disease at all these three levels. For this holistic approach, we have to rely more on alternative systems of medicine. If found beneficial, we should integrate these systems with the modern medicine. Many times in common illnesses, these alternative systems can offer better results. If treated in a holistic way in the beginning, many acute health problems can be cured safely, gently, naturally and more economically. I believe more than 80% of common acute problems can be dealt effectively or perhaps even better by holistic approach. No doubt malnutrition, poverty, uncleanliness, illiteracy contribute a great deal to the ill health of the society. However, pollution, mental stresses, struggle for survival, improper food habits, unhealthy mental attitudes are also responsible for a great majority of chronic health problems.

Allopathic medicine is getting more and more technologically oriented. These innovations have dramatically increased the cost of modern medicine as well as fuelled the expectations of the people. Per capita average expenditure on health has become benchmark of the quality of health care of a nation. More a nation spends on medical care; more developed it is supposed to be. There is an obsession on medical break-through in public mind. Television and other media are full of such exciting medical news. Average person now things that any and every health problem can be fixed with the help of the medical technology.

Stem Cell Research:
Stem Cell research and Human Genome Project are the most recent advances of medicine. Stem Cell Research can probably be translated as " Deliberate destruction of human embryos for the potential benefit of others. " The argument that this research is going to cure many chronic diseases like diabetes, Alzheimer's, arthritis, cancer etc is one sided. It should be noted that majority of chronic diseases are not due to faulty genes. In great majority, these diseases are due to our faulty life styles, improper food, negative thoughts, environmental pollution etc. Improper life styles trigger various diseases, albeit through altered genetic mechanism. Changing genes in few select individuals by gene therapy is not going to fulfill our dream of "Health For All" by 2005 or

2010 etc. Even if the gene therapy helped some select individuals temporarily, the "genetic problems" could soon recur if no corrections of faulty life styles were done. There are many billions populating the earth. The sermons about importance of healthy life styles, healthy diet, attitudes and exercise (which could prevent many chronic diseases) are not very exciting and are usually neglected. These are certainly not as popular as the "Medical Breakthroughs " reported on the national news networks in the prime time news. Gene therapy will NOT be a panacea for all our health problems.

What Is Life?

There is, however, another angle to the stem cell research. The basic question is "When and how does the human life begin?" Visible physical body is NOT the whole human being. We all have subtle invisible body (astral body), which is the seat of our mind, thought and spirit. Physical body dies but this astral body goes through many births, one after another, reaping the fruits of good and bad deeds performed in earlier lives. There are thousands of verified true stories about near death experience, out of body experience, memories of previous births etc. What do these stories indicate?

Seymour Kirlian, a Russian scientist in 1940s, developed a technique to photograph subtle energy body surrounding living being. Kirlian photography is available in US and Europe in various centers. A true scientist should not be prejudiced and should look at the evidence from all the sources. Actual photographs taken with Kirlian technique would suggest that astral body is a real thing and not a fiction of some religious imagination. Astral body is the precursor of physical human body. It is the source of further development of physical body. Any seed is a potential tree, so is an embryo a potential human. Even an embryo having only few cells has a corresponding astral body, with all its emotions and thoughts in a seed form, awaiting manifestation. The life starts with fertilization of an egg! Do we have the right to compel another human life to sacrifice for our ill health, for which we ourselves are largely responsible? Do we have the right to suspend the animation in the human embryos by freezing in our labs? We should not be forced to choose between science and ethics. Our science should be ethical. Science should respect ethics. Only such science can usher true prosperity and peace.

Human Genome Project:

Human Genome mapping is another such break-through. After the unfolding of the human genome recently, we are told that any disease now can be fixed by simply replacing the responsible gene! This is a very distant and probably unrealistic dream. No doubt various diseases are associated with certain genetic abnormalities. Some people are born with genetic weakness and develop certain diseases. However, most of the times, we ourselves have caused this genetic abnormality over the long periods of the time. With our faulty life styles and food habits, we do precipitate many of these conditions. Without attending to basic laws of health, tinkering with genes might prove to be a misdirected attempt to take care of health problems of billions and billions inhabiting this earth. Even after genetic fixing, if such a person continues to ignore the natural laws of health, he or she would soon land up in some other "genetic problem" ready for another "genetic transplant". More and more human embryos will be manufactured in the in the laboratories, ready to supply of the increasing demands of the genes required by the consumers. Only a select few rich people can afford such a treatment. No doubt, medical industry will thrive on such technological advances. Medical scientists will play The God! The gap between haves and have-nots will keep widening.

Future Trends:

It is difficult to foresee where the modern medicine will take us in the next few decades. If the current trends continue, medicine will get more and more technology dependent. Human body will be considered only as an aggregate of material organs that could be fixed, replaced or altered at will. The mind, which animates the physical body, might be ignored. However, there are signs of a new awareness rapidly surging in large sections of society. Modern medicine is very effective in management of trauma, accidents, infections, and emergencies. On the other hand, it is very ineffective and probably bad for treating various chronic degenerative diseases, cancer, allergies, auto-immune diseases, mental diseases, environmental toxic diseases, functional diseases and all those conditions where mind-spirit complex plays an active role in creating such diseases. When this public awareness reaches a critical mass, we are bound to see dramatic changes in our ways of treating diseases.

There are many conditions, which the modern medicine can treat efficiently. One should take all the help from modern medicine in such conditions. However, in the condition where the modern medicine is not effective, one should seek for the evidence based alternative treatments. Many times, selected complementary treatments can be integrated with the modern medicine for optimal results.

The Medical Science is on the verge of radical changes in the near future. Man will be compelled to explore holistic ways to look after the health of humanity. Man will have to tap the internal strength of the mind and the spirit to achieve better health, happiness and peace.

CHAPTER 3

CHRONIC DISEASES

Disease means Loss of Ease! Normal life should be easy, comfortable, and painless; without any anxiety or depression. One should feel happy and fulfilled. The body should be in working order and mind should be joyous and spirit peaceful! Whenever mind and body suffer, that is called the disease. Perception of the suffering is through the mind. When one is fast asleep, there is no awareness of disease or suffering. Body is a miraculous machine and the moment something goes wrong, the brain gets the signals through the elaborate network of the nerves. The mind then becomes aware of the disease.

Diseases can be classified in various ways. A disease could be acute or chronic. A disease could be congenital, right from the birth or could be acquired later on. A disease could be as a result of accident, infection or new growth, which can result in a tumor. A disease could be physical, mental or a combination of both. A disease could be in early stage or in a late stage. A disease could be functional or organic. In functional disease, a person suffers but there may not be any abnormal laboratory tests to document the cause of the suffering. In organic disease, various laboratory tests, X rays, scans etc point to the abnormalities in the body. We are going to look into the causes of diseases.

Acute Illness:
An acute disease appears to start suddenly without much of a warning. However, there is usually an underlying disturbance, which is either neglected or not noticed by the person who becomes victim of the acute precipitation of the medical problem. Acute disease makes the patient bedridden for short period, till he or she gets over or under. Modern medicine has progressed tremendously to take care of acute process of the disease. Emergency surgery can take care of many acute surgical problems. Acute pains due to stones in kidney, gall bladder can be relieved by surgery. Obstructions in the intestines can be corrected.

Heart attacks due to narrowing of blood vessels can be relieved by the bypass. Internal bleedings in brain, abdomen or chest, can be arrested. Intensive Care Units and Coronary Care Units help a lot of patients to recover and survive. Orthopedic surgeries in accidents are very important to save the lives and to make the body functional. In acute infections, antibiotics work wonders. All these acute interventions have glorified medicine. In the television serials, these advances are highlighted and that is what makes a TV serial or a movie thrilling! People get wonderstruck by these images. The idea that modern doctor can fix each and every problem all the time gets engraved in the observers mind. Doctors are looked up with awe and the hospitals are considered to be the temples of the health. However, there is also another side to this picture.

Art of Medicine:
Medicine is not an exact science like mathematics, physics or engineering. Doctors deal with living human beings who have their own minds, attitudes, strengths and weaknesses. If you take your car to a garage, the mechanic can clean the carburetor, tune up engine, change the plugs, service it and the car is ready to be driven. The human body is not like an inert machine, which can be fixed up only mechanically. Body has got a mind that feels; intelligence that knows. Mechanical fixing may not be adequate solution every time. Doctors can prescribe medicines but the body has to heal itself, with the help of the mind and the spirit. Healing comes from within. Patient has to be an equal partner in his or her own healing process. It is not the job of the doctors alone to cure the disease. Without the cooperation and determination of the patients, medicine does not go very far on the way to recovery. Doctors can arrest the symptoms of certain diseases by quick-fixing medicines but one has to go to the root cause of the disease if health is to be restored. If one is not able to address to the root cause of a disease, the acute process is at risk to become a chronic disease.

As stated earlier, human body is a miraculous machine. It is able to self-correct and self maintain, most of the times. Many a times, symptoms like fever, cough, cold, diarrhea, vomiting, spasms, pains could be the warnings of internal disturbance. These are like traffic signals on the road to warn you of the road conditions. These symptoms should not be looked at as enemies but as the warnings of incoming diseases. The symptoms are crying for your attention to the underlying health problem. If a baby is crying due to discomfort, you should see what is bothering the baby. It is no use only to stop the crying forcibly with your hand on the baby's mouth. The symptoms of a disease should be corrected but not unduly suppressed by quick-fixing medicines. Arresting such symptoms too soon may be counterproductive.

Chronic Diseases:

In recent times, the names such diabetes, blood pressure, angina, arthritis, rheumatism, migraine, fatigue, indigestion, acidity, colitis, cancer, irritable moods, anxiety, depression etc have become household words. Chronic diseases are increasing at an alarming rate. Increased life expectancy is a partial explanation for this observation. In old age, many illnesses are likely to affect the body. After all, the body is not immortal. It has to die, some day. As with an old car or old machine, breakdowns are bound to occur as the body gets older. However, this cannot be the whole explanation for rapid increase in chronic diseases. If we look at the world today, there is tremendous increase in pollution. Air we breathe, water we drink, foods we eat usually contain a lot of toxic products. Our bodies are constantly bombarded with toxins in air, water and food. Furthermore, there are subtle toxins that are created within our body with our unhealthy emotions and mental actions. Lack of proper sleep prevents natural repair of the overworked body tissues. Toxins and stress diminish our immunity, disease fighting power.

Toxic Pollution:

There are various toxic and waste products invading our bodies, day and night. Mainly, there are internal toxins and the external toxins. The body itself produces internal waste products. These waste products and toxins are products of our own metabolic process. When our digestive fire is poor, even normal food we eat get incompletely digested. When such products circulate in body, these get lodged in various parts of the body. Ayurved has termed such toxic products as " Aama". The aama, if not digested properly, accumulates and can obstruct the transport of essential nutrients to various parts of the body. Under normal circumstances, liver, intestine, lung, kidneys and skin help the body to dispose toxic waste products. These systems, if overloaded and overworked, slowly fail in their job of keeping the body pure and in good health. If aama accumulates in joints and muscles, arthritis and rheumatism may result. If it accumulates in lungs, one may get respiratory diseases like bronchitis, infections, allergies etc. Aama blocking can lead to circulatory conditions, digestive problems, fevers, and many other conditions. Aama can be reduced by improving digestive power with herbs, exercise, occasional fasting and eating good quality fresh foods. Fast foods, stale foods, fried foods, canned foods, pop drinks, bleached floor and white sugar are hard to digest and usually increase the internal toxins. As a result of metabolism, these foods also create free radicals in the cells, which damage cellular enzyme function and interfere with our health. Free radicals and oxidative damage to our tissues is a big factor leading to chronic ill health. Later on this book, the role of free radicals in relation with cancer will be explained in more details.

We are subjected to innumerable external toxins in the environment. We breathe such toxins in air. Burning of industrial chemicals, petrol, diesel, kerosene etc pollutes the air. To increase the yield of food grains, vegetables and fruits, heavy amounts of synthetic fertilizers, pesticides and insecticides are showered on the crops. Many of these chemicals get mixed with the foods we eat. These enter our body and settle down in different parts of the body. Industrial waste products, containing mercury, lead and similar poisonous minerals find their way into crops as well as in the fish and fowl we eat. Cows, chicken and other farm animals are subjected to heavy use of antibiotics to get more quantity of foods! Mad cow disease recently rocked the European nations. Green revolution has certainly increased the food production but the quality of the foods we are made to consume has become unhealthy. Commercial interests have subjugated the quality food productions. We are urged to use various cosmetic products to look beautiful. Some of these unnatural products could actually harm the body in the long run by blocking our natural cleansing processes.

Invisible Pollution:
Equally important, and perhaps more harmful to our health, are subtle toxins we cannot see. Noise pollution, Electro-magnetic waves, Microwaves, Ionizing Solar Radiations due to breakdown in Ozone Shield of the earth, Radio and Television waves, Cell-phone and Mobile Phone Waves, Geopathic radiations in certain places are just a few examples of such subtle agents, which might affect our health adversely. There are now thousands and thousands of different electrical and electro-magnetic signals simultaneously crowding our air. The atmosphere is loaded with such radiations. We do not exactly know to what extent these invisible waves and noise pollution can impair our health. Although we can not see these radiations, their effects on our instruments are for all to see. Can we dismiss these waves as harmless? These things have changed our lifestyles and made our material life more pleasurable and convenient. Instant communications is a great help for industry, commerce and even for pleasurable recreations in life. In the current age, one cannot imagine a life without all these advances. However, all these subtle pollutants do affect our subtle invisible body. As good music elevates our moods, bad noise pollution can certainly cause emotional and mental irritability. Same is true for various other types of radiations mentioned earlier. Incessant exposures to such subtle atmospheric toxins can harm our health and peace over the long run. Conventionally, a toxin is a chemical substance, which can harm the body. However, we can also term these subtle invisible atmospheric influences as Subtle Toxins since these are able to interfere with the working of our subtle bodies.

Different diseases are thought to be results of separate causes. However, there appears to be a common underlying denominator for a majority of chronic diseases. The incessant attack by the toxins on our bodies slowly weakens our immune system. The toxins get lodged in our various organs. These organs can no longer function normally. At a certain stage, the organ no longer copes and then it rebels. The rebellion gives various symptoms, which we label as different diseases. We try to treat and suppress these symptoms. The disease process goes deeper in body and this is the start of a chronic disease. Deeper it goes; more difficult it is to cure.

Genetic Changes:
Although toxins are same, the expressions of disease will be as per the individual susceptibility. Due to proper life styles, habits and perhaps hereditary strength, many people would be able to cope up with incessant attacks of pollutants. However, some others might start loosing the battle, sooner or later. These toxins can also slowly alter the genes by mutations and start specific chronic diseases like diabetes, blood pressure, colitis, cancer, arthritis etc. Personal manifestation of a disease mainly depends upon that person's genetic susceptibility. It must be stated again that genetic abnormality is not always something you are born with. Although, one can be born with certain genetic disorders, many times original genes can slowly change due to mutation as result of improper life styles and exposure to toxins.

There would be a lot of arguments about the validity of these observations. However, these points are well proved scientifically in many recent laboratory experiments. To speak about cancer, the existence of some genes, termed as oncogenes, has been proved under microscope. Further, these oncogenes either prevent cancer or cause cancer depending upon some external stimulations. The same friendly gene, which prevents cancer in healthy state, can be turned on to start cancer. When activated by prolonged exposure to carcinogenic substances as tobacco, chemicals, tar products, certain pharmaceuticals etc, the same gene causes cancer growth! The same is true for many other chronic disease conditions.

Detoxification of Body:
No doubt, some diseases in childhood as well as later on in adult life are due to inherited genes. However, onset of a specific disease can be usually delayed due to proper precautions and life style changes. One should note that one is mainly responsible for one's own health, either good or bad. If you get any disease condition, you yourself are an

important partner in your own treatment. Proper awareness of natural health laws and adherence to good habits would go a long way in making you healthier!

Fortunately, we might be able to remove these accumulated toxins from the body by various means. Intestines, kidneys, lung, liver, skin etc, the natural detoxification channels of the body, can be strengthened. Special detoxification techniques can be used to accelerate the process of purification. Ayurveda recommends Pancha-karma; five fold purification, for detoxification and purification of the tissues. Homeopathic remedies and many herbal preparations are known to promote detoxification process. Chelation has been used in some special circumstances for reducing toxic deposits in body. Even regular exercise, occasional fasting, controlling diet, taking proper vitamins and mineral supplements, meditation, yoga, relaxation are known to promote detoxification. If one has to treat chronic diseases effectively, these points should be addressed primarily.

CHAPTER 4.

Causes of Cancer

Cancer is a common, controversial and confusing condition. We need not give any statistics to prove that Cancer is getting commoner in this age. After having spent billions and billions of dollars in the past few decades on cancer research, the world has not yet found concise cause or comfortable cure for cancer. The time has finally come to look into a different direction for the truth.

Cancer disease was known to the people of ancient times. Sushrut Samhita, an Ayurvedic text dating back to 700 B.C. mentions tumor diseases by various categories such as arbuda, granthi, vidradhi, gulma etc. Kark-Roga, which is a translation of the English term cancer, is not an Ayurvedic term. . Hippocrates, a Greek physician (400 B.C.), was the first physician to name this disease as Carcinoma- (karkinoma: Greek word for crab), since he found it spreading like a crab. The name "Cancer ", which means crab, came in routine use later on. Traces of cancer have been found even in the bones of Egyptian mummies embalmed 5000 years ago. The cancer is becoming more and more common and has become like an epidemic disease of the modern times. In the developed countries, it is the second commonest cause of death, second only to heart disease.

Cancer is due to chaos in the rational biology. Cancer starts when healthy cells stop functioning and maturing properly. A mishap occurs within the cells. It probably begins with a genetic change (mutation) of the DNA, which is the part of nucleus of the cell. DNA is the material out of which chromosomes and genes are made. DNA has the property of automatic duplication to create new cells. Old cells, when no longer needed by the body, mature and die. These cells are replaced by new young cells by a process of cell division called mitosis. Life mechanism in a healthy body can control the rate of growth and destruction of cells precisely as per the needs. There is perfect balance in Creator and

Destroyer principles. Mutations do occur even normally but very rarely. These mutations are repaired and the cycle goes on. Due to persistent exposure of the tissues to abnormal irritation, either internally or externally, rate of mutation goes beyond control. DNA, the blueprint of the cells, turns abnormal and starts producing abnormal cells. This is the beginning of cancer. Even at this stage, cancer like cells are routinely eliminated by healthy immune system. When immunity fails, cancer can grow unchallenged and result is a visible tumor.

Theories About Cancer:
There are numerous theories to explain what causes cancer. It is an intriguing subject. No final answer has been yet reached. One single theory is unable to explain the causation of all types of cancers. Cancer may not be one single disease, although the end product of the disease process appears as a visible tumor or ulcer. As suggested above, the final event is the escape of the cell cycle from the natural control system of the body called immunity. Immunity is a complex system and there are various facets to immunity. Immunity can be selectively disturbed to cause a specific disease such as cancer, arthritis, infections, AIDS etc. Following are some theories about cancer.

1. **"Wish Theory ":** This is a fundamental assumption to analyze the personality of an individual that might invite cancer, unknowingly! Modern medicine now appreciates the "Power of Mind over Matter", which has always been the basic belief of holistic medical sciences, philosophy, theosophy, yoga etc. Here a person's attitude towards life is a critical factor. A person may subconsciously feel that the life is not worth living. Cancer might be one of the escape routes. A person might sincerely feel that "Life has become purposeless", "Life has become miserable", "Life has become a burden", "There is no hope", " Nobody loves me", "No one wants me", "Its no use" etc. Psychological distress can find a physical outlet such as cancer or some other chronic disease. About 20% of all the cancer patients fall in this group. These patients subconsciously or even consciously wish to die and welcome cancer or some other

serious illness as an escape route. Another 60 % patients are in middle group that will follow the doctor's orders without any questions. They do not wish to discuss about their disease and about what more can be done to overcome the cancer. They would accept the treatment and its outcome passively, whatever that might be. The last 20% patients are fighters. They are optimistic and eager to beat their cancer, at any cost. They would ask many questions, explore various options and would participate in their own health care. It is in this last group of optimist activists that the chances for cancer cure are very high.

There are various shades of negative feelings about one's own life. After retirement a person, unable to switch to other hobbies or occupations, might feel life as purposeless. An elderly woman might feel that she is no longer needed by her family and might loose interest in own life. Death of spouse or loved ones sometimes produces long lasting unresolved grief. In old age, death of husband or wife is especially traumatic. Neglect by own children in old age is very stressful. Life becomes miserable and worthless. Unexpected losses in business and reversal of fortune are other events hard to cope up with. This may be one reason why cancer is common in old age, when one has weathered many a storms in life. Not everyone who experiences such bad events would have health problems. It is not the event itself but how a person reacts to it is more important.

Feeling of rejection can produce stress. Person's willpower to live might be destroyed by stressful events. Finally, the mind sends signals to body. The switch to "desire for life" is subconsciously turned off. Mind is all-powerful, like the *kalpavriksha*- wish fulfilling tree! It eventually grants you whatever you wish for, either good or bad. The body gets the message and obeys. Immunity on the cell level gets affected and cancer takes roots. Recently, direct nerve links were discovered from brain to thymus and spleen. Thymus and spleen play a very important role in immunity. Right signals from the brain can improve immunity while wrong signals can destroy it. Under chronic stress, brain sends harmful signals and immunity is reduced. All this happens subconsciously. The person or the relatives are not aware. Only good thing about this is that the person can help himself or herself if he or she is able to consciously reverse this negative process by positive thoughts, affirmations and changes in the attitude. It is a hard job but worth trying, for our own sake. Meditation, yoga, prayers, social support and striving for some goal in life are the ways to do this job right. Optimistic patient with positive attitude usually succeeds in the battle.

2. **"Diet Theory"**: Nutrition is critical. Good nutrition can prevent cancer and conversely poor nutrition can invite cancer. In the past 10 years, a lot of research has been done on various minerals, vitamins, amino acids, fatty acids, polysaccharides, enzymes and other natural substances, which have cancer preventive properties. The details of this will be explained later.

3. **Genetic Theory**: Inborn weakness in certain genes, called oncogenes, can make some people prone to get certain types of cancers more frequently than average. Cancer of breast, colon and ovary appears to be more common in blood relatives. It is estimated that less than 10 % of cancers are due to inborn genetic weakness. In a way this is good news, which means that more than 90% cancers are not due to hereditary cancer risk genes. Even if parents, siblings or other relatives have cancer, one still doesn't have very high chance for getting cancer. Cancer risk can be greatly reduced by healthy life style and proper nutrition, even if one is born with cancer prone genes. Avoidance of outside causes that trigger cancer would further help to reduce such risk. Most of the times, cancer starts after acquired genetic mutations, which are due to exposures to carcinogens in later life. It is in our hands to reduce such risks further by healthy life styles, which will be described later in the chapters on the treatment of cancer.

4. **"Chemical, Physical and Biological Carcinogens"**: Numerous pollutants, chemicals, toxins that are so common in the

environment can trigger cancer in some people. Smoking and chewing tobacco are most widely publicized hazards. Certain drugs are also known to cause cancer. X-rays, gamma rays and ultraviolet rays are known to cause certain types of cancers. Geopathic radiations from earth at certain locations, adverse magnetic and electrical fields, and noise pollution are some other physical causes, which could increase the risk of cancer. Biological materials such as certain viruses are associated with cancer. A virus is a small fragment of DNA or RNA, which can easily enter into the nucleus of cells. Some viruses can "infect" and convert the normal genetic code of the cells into cancer mode. This process turns the affected cells cancerous. Virus is linked with certain types of lymph node cancers, warts and cancer of uterus.

5. **"Toxic Dump Theory"**: As a house needs cleaning, the body needs a safe disposal system for waste products and toxins. In good health, organs like liver, intestines, kidneys, skin and lungs are doing the function of the waste disposal. If these organs are not efficient or if the waste products are too much to handle, there is accumulation of toxic waste products in the body. Some doctors believe that body creates tumors as a dumping ground for toxic wastes. Removing a tumor without reducing toxic load and without repairing the sanitary team of the body, might not lead to permanent control. The continued flow of waste products would need to search for other places in the body to act as a dumping ground. This might be what we call as a recurrence or metastasis of cancer.

6. **"Rebellion Theory"**: After chronic abuse of our own body with unhealthy habits and improper lifestyles, certain organs in body might feel neglected. We neglect the needs of such organs. The owner of the body ignores all the warning signals by such organs. The miracle machine, that is our body, which was given to us free of charge with lifetime warranty, starts deteriorating. Eventually, some cells, tissues and organs declare the war,

overthrowing all the central controls. The cells start growing in chaos and soon cancer tumor is formed.

7. **Childhood Cancer:** This is a very special subject. It is very hard for the parents to see infants and young children victim of cancer. The whole family is shattered. The image of suffering child, due to cancer and due to treatment reactions, is heartbreaking for the close relatives. Young children are oblivious to the impact of the diagnosis but faced with repeated pains of injections, most of them develop deep fears about the doctors and hospitals. Later on, if the condition starts deteriorating and pain becomes a major problem for a small child, all feel greatly hurt.

These children never had time to smoke, develop bad lifestyles or indulge in any other unhealthy activities. Why then the God is giving such punishment to an innocent little human? Such occasions are very traumatic for the relatives of the child and for the medical staff treating the child. I have observed that most of the times, such little patients have a divine aura and innocent look. We feel hopeless and desperate that we are unable to give much medical help except for kind words and cheers. This often makes us cry internally.

Apart from the theory of inherited genetic weakness, it is possible that pregnant mothers might have been exposed to carcinogens and toxins during the pregnancy. These toxins easily cross the placenta in the uterus and are able to exert bad effects on the growing fetus very easily. That is why a pregnant woman's behavior, diet, medication and moods are so important for the unborn baby. Women subjected to drugs, smoking, toxic medications, domestic quarrels, stress etc are known to give birth to babies who later on develop various diseases.

In childhood, rapidly growing cancers e.g. kidney cancer, neuroblastoma of nerves, retinoblastoma of eyes, leukemia of blood etc are common. These cancers might have a short latent period of few months to couple of years as opposed to adult cancers that need exposures of 10 to 15 years or even longer to "sprout the seeds of cancer" within the body. Secondly, karma theory, destiny etc, which is explained below might play a part in childhood cancers

8. **Metaphysical Influence Theory:** Although not yet accepted by current scientific logic, certain locations in some houses are observed to cause to chronic ill health to the occupants of such locations. This could be due to certain negative elements influencing certain locations. Changing the houses or changing positions of sleeping etc have resolved chronic health problems in certain people. Current scientific instruments cannot measure these subtle influences. However many spiritual healers, vastu-shastris, saints and yogis can perceive these subtle influences. Astrological predictions about health problems would come in the same category.

9. **"Karma Theory":** When nothing else explains a disease, one has to go to Hindu concept of *Karma*, deeds performed either in this life or in past lives. "As you sow, so shall you reap" is the thought not only of Hindu religion but many other religions have similar concepts. Cancer in very young infants or children, who could not have got the "chance" to get exposed to carcinogens, bad diet etc could be explained by such assumptions. Saints like Lord Gautam Buddha, Ramakrishna Paramahansa, Raman Maharshi, Swami Akhandanand Saraswati etc are some examples of divine souls who developed cancer at the end. Such incidences cannot be explained by any other theories. One could call this The Divine Will.

Cancer As Terrorist Attack:

Cancer can perhaps be seen as a Terrorist Attack on the body. This vision has become even more pertinent after the events of September

11th in New York and later on at the Indian Parliament on December 13th 2001. These events were the eye-openers to the whole world. This was like a confirmed diagnosis of cancer after the surgical biopsy! Minor troubles in various parts of the world for the past many decades were looked upon as local skirmishes, which would somehow be settled through "Peaceful Negotiations" This was a politically correct attitude, which is usually to push chronic problems under the carpet. (Please note: I am not against any dialogues or negotiated settlements of any problems. I am all for it. This should be our first line of action. But sometimes one needs to follow the dialogues and protests with the ACTION. Hindu moral codes have prescribed 4 levels of responses to overcome unpleasant situations: Saama, Daama, Danda and Bheda, in that order) When America was under direct attack, the world community acknowledged the diagnosis of the Terrorist Cancer affecting the whole world. It was no longer a local complaint.

Bombing the Terrorists:
This had to be dealt with severe blows to the terrorist hideouts around the world. The fireworks started in Afghanistan to destroy the terrorists. The world community swore to chase and destroy the last surviving terrorist to make the world terror free. It was not convenient to pay attention to the basic issues why and how the terrorists were created.
The current approach is " First destroy the terrorists and then the world would be automatically become the same comfortable place to live and enjoy the pleasures of life." Bombing the terrorist camps is much easier than to resolve any festering chronic regional disputes! Latter proposition is much more difficult to achieve. It requires long-term commitment, sacrifice and fairness. Can you see the simile in Terrorist Problem and Cancer Problem? The terrorist problem affects the whole world. The cancer problem affects whole body. In human cancer, we try to chase and destroy the last surviving cancer cell in our body, with our firepower- radiation, chemotherapy or radical surgery. The damage to innocent civilian population is accepted as " Co-lateral Damage"! After the fireworks, we doctors feel that somehow the patient will be all right since we have removed or destroyed all the visible terror of cancer. Unless attention is given to rehabilitation of the whole body with

correction of causative factors, the threat of recurrence of cancer persists.

Carcinogens:
Carcinogen is a chemical or physical agent that can cause cancer. Mere exposure to carcinogen does not guarantee the onset of cancer. However, such exposures increase the risk of getting cancer. If such exposures were avoided, it would reduce the risk of cancer. There are hundreds of known carcinogens; many more yet remain unknown. We have not fully understood all the causes and mechanisms of cancer. What we have got are various theories. All such theories have some truths but each theory would be unable to explain the totality of cancer problem. One thing is definite; cancer risk increases due to long term attack of carcinogens on the body. How do these carcinogen spark the onset of cancer is still a mystery.

To put it very simply, fire cannot start with matchsticks alone or with a can of petrol alone. As long as these two do not come in contact with each other, there is no fire. The moment both these things are ready, fire starts easily. Soil and seed theory of cancer suggests that your body is the soil where the seed of cancer can grow. If the soil is not ready, seed of cancer will not grow. Even if the soil is ready but if cancer seeds (carcinogens) are avoided, risk of cancer can be greatly reduced. We do not know all the seed types of cancer. Cancer cannot be 100 % prevented even if we follow a healthy life style. However, the chances of cancer will be greatly reduced. To take care of the soil, that is our body, is mostly in our hands. About the seeds, sometimes we are helpless or in the dark.

Oncogenes:
The recent genetic research has discovered specific genes in the cells, which are called oncogenes. These genes can either cause cancer or prevent cancer. These genes are parts of chromosomes, which forms the nucleus of individual cells in body. It is hard to see how same gene can prevent cancer on one hand and also promote it on the other hand. How can a same gene be so much different at different times? We should

remember that many things have duel purpose in life. A door can be used either to allow a friend in the house or to throw out an enemy. It is not the fault of the door. It is the user who is responsible for the use of the door. Therefore it is no big surprise to see that the same oncogene can either prevent cancer or trigger the cancer depending upon the user of the gene that is your body and mind.

Here lies the importance of nature's laws of health, good life styles, and healthy food for body and for mind. Elevate your spirit to grant yourself the peace and the happiness, which is your birthright. Lokamanya Tilak said, " Independence is My Birth Right!" This proclamation should not be taken only in the political context, which is apt to be distorted and twisted for selfish motives of some groups in the society. With the rights come the responsibilities. We all love to have rights but who wants the responsibilities! The responsibility is for others while the rights are exclusively mine, thus thinks the human mind. This is the basic cause of unrest, injustice and fights of the world. When our organs start fighting against each other, neglecting the welfare of the entire person, same situation arises. Whatever is in Brahmanda it is in Pinda. Whatever is in macrocosm, it is in microcosm. Man is the Holographic image of the entire Universe!

Immunity and Cancer:
Continuous Irritation of some part of our body, over many years, could start cancer process. The actual period required to trigger onset of cancer varies greatly from person to person. In some persons it might take 15 to 20 years, while in some others it could be as short as few months. No definite rules exist to predict this. It is known that cancer like cells are sometimes found in perfectly healthy individuals. These cells are caught and destroyed by healthy immune system before they establish and multiply. This is natural cancer prevention, which happens routinely in most of us. Our immune system, consisting of white blood cells- lymphocytes, natural killer cells, interleukins, interferon, mast cells, macrophages etc is like efficient police force in a city.

The immune cells are constantly on the lookout for disease producing germs and abnormal cells. These cells work round the clock, day and night, without any rest or leave. The immune cells are constantly being replenished. As old cells die new cells are formed and recruited. These immune cells seek, identify, encircle, attack and eventually destroy the enemy cells and germs. Thus, our health is maintained. In infections, germs overpower us temporarily. An active immune system soon enlists more immune cells to fight the battle, which is won in a few days. This acute process is accompanied by fever and other symptoms of infection. Fever is the result of the infection rather than the cause of the infection. Symptoms are like road signs to warn you about the road conditions during your journey. Hasty use of medicines to quickly reduce fever is sometimes counterproductive. Fever is the war cry of the body expressing the internal fight. This is an open war.

Cancer is usually secret war. This is due to secret activities of terrorists, which are not noticed quickly by NOT SO EFFICIENT police force that is our low immunity. This is so called " Failure of Intelligence"! Cancer like cells are allowed to grow and expand their activities. Our neglect of natural health laws even encourages the formation of cancer cells. Let us now review some of the external cancer causing materials, which are called carcinogen. These promote cancer in a body, which is weakened due to genetic alterations and from accumulation of toxic waste products in the cells.

Some Common Carcinogens

PHYSICAL	CHEMICAL	NUTRITIONAL
1.Sunlight- Ultraviolet rays	1.Polluted Water	1.Diet deficiencies
2.Electro-magnetic Fields	2.Chlorinated Water	2.Toxins due to metabolism
3.Geopathic Stress	3.Fluoridated Water	3. Intestinal toxicity
4.Nuclear Radiations	4.Tobacco products	4. Digestive impairment
	5.Pesticides	
BIOLOGICAL	6.Food Additives	**EMOTIONAL**
1.Viruses,	7.Tar & Petroleum Products	1.Chronic stress
2.Parasites	8.Certain drugs	2.Toxic negative emotions

Food as a Cause of Cancer?
We would be surprised even to imagine that food, which all of us are eager to eat everyday, could lead to cancer! Is it possible? Let us think more in this matter. No doubt, food is what keeps the world going. Without food all the life would perish. Food is the raw material, which is supplied to create the final products i.e. healthy cells, tissues, organs etc. The food is also used for energy, which is essential for all the activities. Compare this with a factory. Raw materials are being used to produce goods. If the quality of the raw material is inferior, you don't expect the finished products to be good! If the food we eat is deficient in the essential elements, the body cannot function properly. Health would be affected for sure. This may not be obvious immediately, but over the years, the bad effects would be obvious. Nowadays, most of the foods we eat are contaminated with chemicals, pollutants, germs, pesticides and insecticides. If proper precautions are not taken to wash off such products before preparation of the food, these pollutants enter our body. The risk of eating contaminated, stale, unclean food is even higher, when we eat out in restaurants.

In the past few years, a detailed research has been done on Nutrition and Health. It has been proved that quality of the food, vegetables and fruits is extremely important either for keeping good health. Bad quality leads to bad health! All the essential vitamins, minerals, fatty acids, amino acids etc are naturally found in fresh vegetables, fruits, grains, nuts and dairy products. Vitamin C is an important anti-oxidant that prevents damage due to free radicals in the body. Vitamin E is essential for purification and for healthy cell function. Vitamin B-Complex is essential for actions of various enzymes, which regulate all the chemical activities in the body at cellular levels. The body needs sufficient amounts of minerals like zinc, selenium, magnesium, manganese, calcium, phosphorus, potassium to prevent cancer and other diseases. Co-enzyme Q-10 is needed to prevent cancer and to promote normal heart function.

There are many other essential food elements linked with good health. The deficiency of these would obviously lead to increased risk of cancer. In the olden days, all these requirements were usually met through consumption of fresh, clean, locally grown food. In the modern days of commercial food technology, practices of food canning, freezing, food irradiation, hybrid seeds etc are getting popular. Good quality foods are vanishing. Pasteurized, homogenized, refrigerated milk is more difficult to digest and less healthy than the fresh milk locally produced and freshly consumed.

It may not be possible to turn the clock back and go to olden ways of living. However, reader should at least be aware of the merits and demerits of eating various types of foods in this modern age. Aerated pop drinks, like cola, soda etc, are known to cause health problems in the long run. Refined foods such as white sugar, bakery products, and white bread are known to cause digestive problems in a many people. When you are healthy and when your digestive power is strong in young age, these foods cause no immediate damage. In the long run, consumption of foods deficient in nutritional quality is likely to lead to various health problems. With proper food habits, one may prevent or delay the onset of cancer. With improper food habits, one may hasten the onset of cancer. This is not only a general comment. Recent research has shown that certain essential elements in nutritional therapy can actually reverse the process of cancer!

Foods That Fight Cancer:
Food is a very important factor for health. Good food can prevent disease and keep you healthy. Bad food can disturb your health and cause disease. In the past 20 years, a lot of research has been done on various food factors. Natural vitamins A, C, B-complex, D and E are shown to reduce risk of cancer. Minerals like Zinc, Selenium, Copper, Manganese, and Magnesium are vital components of enzymes that help the body fight cancer. Essential fatty acids and essential amino acids are needed for healthy body and for prevention of cancer. Most of these items are provided by the Nature in various fresh vegetables, fruits, dairy products and other natural foods. However, it is becoming increasingly difficult to obtain fresh food products that are free from contamination.

The modern farming practices of use of synthetic fertilizers and pesticides have reduced the health quality of many food items available to common man. Animal farming on a commercial scale has reduced the quality of eggs, fish, meats, chicken etc. Besides introducing a lot of chemical preservatives of dubious quality, addition of preservatives in canned foods reduces nutritional value of foods. The current laws "permit" all these additives and food colors, but as more and more data becomes available, these laws might have to be revised. Certain germs and fungi can enter our bodies through foods we eat. Such contaminated foods can increase the risk for cancer.

Toxic Kitchen Cabinet:
Many common household items could be a source of toxins and could contaminate the foodstuff. Plastics, aluminum cookware and household cleaners could provide such toxic contamination, which might lead to cancer in long run. When foods are cooked in aluminum pots, some aluminum compounds may leak into the foods by chemical reactions or

due to high temperature reached during cooking. As far as possible, aluminum cookware should be avoided for cooking foods.

Plastics are being used increasingly in all our life activities and especially for storage of food, water and other liquids. The safety of plastics is controversial. In microwave cooking, the toxic compounds from the plastic containers such as polyethylene chloride (PVC), polyvinylidene chloride (PVDC), polyethylene (PE) and shining plasticizers used in plastic wraps can migrate into food at high temperatures. These tar products are sources of bio-toxicity as well as environmental pollution.

Many dishwashing liquids, bleaches, chlorinated scouring powders contain petrochemical products. All the detergents are absorbed through the skin and if used improperly, can cause ill health. One should be aware of these subtle dangers so common in our every day modern life. Nontoxic safer biodegradable alternatives instead of toxic detergents are becoming available as per the demands of the health conscious public in developed countries.

Internal Metabolic Toxins:
Internal waste products are liberated in the body due to improper digestion and faulty elimination. Overeating puts extra load on our digestive capacity. Incompletely digested food particles do circulate in the blood and lodge in various cells. These toxins are termed as *Aama* by *Ayurved*, which extensively deals with this subject. *Aama* is responsible for various painful and chronic diseases. Various food contaminants eaten with food cannot be eliminated from body and these get stored in various tissues of the body. Toxic metals like mercury and lead are well known examples of accumulated toxins in the body. These can lead to various diseases by interfering with normal enzyme functions. Bad foods work indirectly leading to various diseases, cancer being one of the expressions of bad food habits.

Chemical Toxins:

Tobacco chewing and tobacco smoking are most publicized cancer causing habits. In various scientific studies, use of tobacco is linked with cancer, lung disease, heart disease and stroke. Smoking can cause cancer of lung while tobacco chewing can cause cancer of mouth and lips. Circulation is affected. That is why the government requires the companies to put the statutory warning "Cigarette Smoking Is Injurious to Health"! This warning is put in very small letters at the bottom of big attractive advertisements depicting handsome men being adored by lovely women! Various filters are claimed to reduce the nicotine and tar contents of the product for increased safety for the smokers. Of course, the best thing would be to give up smoking and chewing tobacco. It is claimed, by the cigarette companies, that every adult is able to decide for himself whether or not he should smoke. Why not give up the cigarettes totally with all their filters? The choice is yours.

Gutka eating has similar problems. Harmful chemicals of the tobacco smoke irritate the lining of throat, air-passages and lungs and lead to onset of cancer after many years. If a smoker quits smoking before he gets cancer, his risk of getting cancer is partly reduced. Tobacco chewing also irritates lining of lips and mouth. After many years, small ulcers are formed. These do not heal and soon turn cancerous. There are many other chemicals known to increase the risk of cancer.

Tar products, which are used in industry routinely, are known to promote cancer. Various artificial perfumes and cosmetics are made from tar products and these are potentially harmful. Kerosene, diesel and petrol are oil products in the same family as tar. Pollution due to these products can lead to various chronic diseases and possibly cancer.

There are other industrial chemicals causing cancer, if accidentally inhaled, ingested or applied to the skin. Aniline dyes are one such example. Insecticides and pesticides, which are widely used in agriculture industry, are passed on to consumers who eat grains, vegetables and fruits contaminated with such products. Washing such products before eating reduces the contamination to some extent. However, if these toxic products have entered the food chains, it is not possible to reduce their levels. One has to be careful about what one eats and about how these products are grown.

Many pesticides such as DDT, gamaxine, Orange etc are now banned because of the health hazards, which were discovered only after many years use. Some toxic products are discharged into rivers and lakes. The water is used for drinking. The fish grown in such water is eaten. The water is used for growing crops, grains and vegetables. All such practices are detrimental to health and potentially carcinogenic. There are thousands and thousands of such polluting toxins. Prima facie evidence about the harmful nature of such toxic products should be enough to warn us to stay away from such products. To test each product for cancer will be impracticable and will certainly delay the commonsense conclusions, which are obvious.

There are a lot of pharmaceutical products, which could cause cancer. Ironically, most of the chemotherapy drugs used for the treatment of cancer are known to cause cancer after some years. This warning is clearly written in the product literature supplied with each drug. Obviously, one has to use such drugs to control serious diseases like cancer etc, but great caution should be exercised for the use of many pharmaceutical products. Use of certain hormones like estrogens and androgens is linked with cancers of breast, uterus and prostate. These medicines should be used only under advice and supervision of experienced medical doctors. Some of the pharmaceutical products have damaging effects on liver, kidney, blood, bones stomach, intestines etc. These warnings are described in the medical books and drug literature. Please remember that a drug is a double-edged weapon. It should be used cautiously and properly, only when necessary.

Germs As A Cause of Cancer:
Bacteria, viruses and similar germs are associated with cancer. Papilloma virus is known to cause cancer of the uterus- cervix. A specific virus causes Burkett's Lymphoma, a cancer of lymph nodes. These are only few known associations between germs and cancer. Many germs might be indirectly responsible for cancer. Chronic

infections in mouth, teeth, throat, lungs, abdomen, urinary track, sex organs and other parts of the body cause long-term biological irritation locally. As with any other chronic local irritation, such chronic infections might lead to cancer, if not attended to promptly. Cancer of the Cervix-uterus is a very common cancer comprising 20 % to 30 % of all cancers affecting women in India. This cancer is linked to poor hygiene and multiple pregnancies. Undoubtedly, women undergoing multiple frequent pregnancies are prone to repeated injuries and infections of uterus. This might be the explanation for the high incidence of cancer in such women.

Ayurved describes germs as "*Krumi*". In Ayurvedic Textbooks, krumis are classified as visible and invisible. Krumis are causes of various diseases. More research needs to be done on krumis to see which type of krumis can be linked with cancer. Dr Royal Rife, a prominent doctor from California, did extensive research in 1930s and 1940s on cancer causing germs. As per his research, a germ (which he termed as BX virus) is the cause of most of the cancers. He studied this virus under a high power microscope, specially developed by him. Dr. Rife concluded that BX virus is the cause of most of the cancers and a specific electro-magnetic ray beam could destroy these viruses. These rays are not the X-rays or cobalt rays that are currently used in radiation treatment of cancer.   The rays coming from Rife machines are called Rife Rays. Dr. Rife claimed that he could cure many cancers, without any harmful side effects, by using his electrical therapy. These claims need to be verified and studied further.

Germ Theory Controversy:
 Dr. Enderlein, another scientist from Germany, proved that small viral like innocent live particles are present in all the cells of healthy body. These viral like living particles could be seen only under dark field microscopy of live blood slides. Staining the slides with laboratory chemicals renders the specimen dead and hence these living particles cannot be seen in action under conventional microscopic techniques. Under the influence of unhealthy life styles, these innocent particles, termed as protits, can change into disease producing fungi, bacteria and

viruses. These particles then cause various diseases as per the local conditions in the body. This theory is known as "Theory of Polymorphism" as opposed to the currently popular "Theory of Monomorphism" proposed by Louise Pasteur and his followers in 19th century.

The theory of monomorphism suggests that each infectious disease is caused by a separate germ, while the Enderlein Theory of Polymorphism proposes that different germs can develop from basic innocent living viral-like particles normally present in all living cells! There are hard-line scientific proponents and opponents on both sides of this controversial battle. More research needs to be done to throw light.

Cancer is triggered by long-standing chronic infections in certain people. As per the allopathic medicine, germs of most of the infective agents are not directly linked to cancer. It is possible that chronic infections might reduce the immunity further and make the organs more susceptible for the growth of cancer.

Physical Toxins:
Excessive solar radiations, ultra violet rays and X-rays found in solar rays are known to cause cancer. Skin cancer is especially common in people with white skin living in regions like Australia, New Zealand etc. Fortunately such skin cancers, which are known as basal cell carcinoma of skin, can be treated and cured most of the times with surgical operations. Harmful radiations can come from certain locations on the earth. This is termed as Geopathic Radiation. These invisible rays and magnetic vibrations can affect our health. Even in certain buildings, some locations could be harmful. Changing bed positions away from these mysteriously harmful locations has improved health of many chronically ill patients. This is termed as "Sick Building Syndrome". Although dismissed by some modern scientists as cases of blind faith and coincidences, these changes have helped many people. There are elaborate rules mentioned in Vastu Shastra, Astrology and Magnetic Therapy textbooks dealing with such positions and locations.

There are man made radiations, from X-ray machines, radioactive isotopes and certain electrical machines. These rays, in high dose over long periods, could increase the risk of cancer. There are stringent requirements and controls to manufacture such equipment. However, careful monitoring of adherence to these standards is difficult. Recently, rays coming out from televisions, mobile phones, microwave ovens etc are also being looked upon with suspicion. Researchers are trying to evaluate effects of such radiation on human health. It is a difficult task, especially because people may not accept to live without such gadgets and also because of the commercial interest, which partly influence the outcome of some of the research studies. The controversy will continue in the foreseeable future. At this stage, each individual should weigh the risks and benefits of such gadgets and then decide for him or herself. Noise pollution, which is getting from bad to worse, is detrimental to health. High levels of disturbing noise do produce mental irritability and eventually affects our immunity. With reduced immunity and increased mental tensions, any disease can take hold of the body. Although cancer is not yet linked directly to noise pollution, it is certainly promoting chronic ill health of the masses.

Mechanical Injuries:

Mechanical injuries are known to leave local weakness in the organs of the body. There are many examples of brain tumors, bone tumors and muscle tumors in patients who give history of injury to the affected area few months or few years before the appearance of actual tumor. Modern medicine dismisses any links between injury and cancer, probably because it cannot be 100 % certain about the links! We need not wait till we are 100% certain about whether each risk factor really causes cancer. There are infinite risk factors and it is not possible to be 100 % sure about anything in the life. One has to trust his commonsense and intuition about coming to own conclusions. It is a common experience that whatever is printed in black-and-white may not be always the ultimate truth. Ayurved clearly states that after apparent cure of an illness or injury, some local weakness is left in that particular organ. Ayurved calls this residual weakness as *Khah-Vaigunya*, which literally means " Weakness of Space". Such local weakness stays dormant until other causes trigger a disease. When unhealthy factors affect the body, such weak points are the first to be affected in the expression of the disease. Chewing hard substances like supari might injure gums and teeth. Mechanical frictions and injuries may produce local weakness, increasing the risk for cancer in some persons.

Dental Work as a Cause of Ill health:
Bad broken teeth might cut and irritate your tongue and lips. If these injuries persist over a long period, these can lead to chronic inflammations, infections and perhaps cancer. Dental health of masses has deteriorated in the past few decades. Cavities, root canals, gum infections, tooth abscess have become household words. This epidemic of dental problems may be partly due to the inferior quality of foods we eat. We as a society eat too much white sugar, sweet foods, canned foods, stale foods, soft foods and fast foods. Pollution in food, air and water may be adding to our dental problems. The modern lifestyle may be partly responsible for the dental problems.

Recently a lot of attention is being paid by the practitioners of the alternative medicine to the possible links between dental disease, dental treatments and chronic illnesses. Chinese acupuncture medicine proposes that each tooth is linked, through acupuncture energy channels, (meridians), to different internal organs of the body such as heart, lungs, kidneys, adrenals, liver, spleen, intestine, gall bladder, muscles, joints etc. It is suggested that dental problems may reflect internal diseases and conversely internal diseases may be caused by the dental problems. Mercury-silver amalgam, which was being used to fill the dental cavities, might be a subtle source of chemical toxins. Slow liberation of toxic mercury and silver compound, even in minute amounts, is able to disturb the health of various organs in the body. Root canal treatments, which are so common these days, might be leaving the dead tooth, again a source for chronic infections, behind in its' own place. This might be responsible for many chronic health problems. These are the theories and there are hot arguments between the proponents and opponents of these theories. One has to be aware about such things to chart one's own strategy for better health. After all, your own health is your own responsibility. Doctors can only guide you but either improving your own health or inviting ill health is largely dependent upon your own actions. Doctors can prescribe, but the cure has to come from within you.

Emotional Toxins:
We all easily understand the chemical and physical toxins in the world. However, toxic emotions are equally responsible in creation of health problems. Negative attitudes are generated through emotions like anger, hatred, blaming habits, excessive guilt, unforgiveness, brooding, revenge, aggression, fear, inferiority etc. These emotions are natural to some extent in all of us. However, when excessive and persistent, these negative thoughts can accelerate chronic health problems. In my practice over the past 30 years, I have observed hundreds and hundreds of patients whose cancer disease surfaced after some painful life events. Death of a loved one, loss of job, painful domestic relations, sudden financial problems, unexpected disappointments, bad turns of fortune etc somehow trigger the process of cancer. Conversely, overcoming these difficulties with positive mental attitude can help a lot in the control of cancer.

Bad mental tendencies (*Vaasana- called shad-ripu*: six enemies in Sanskrit) are creating havoc in the world through their subtle destructive satanic powers. Unhealthy passions, anger, greed, delusion, egotistic pride and jealousy are the six enemies, which harm the person himself who harbors these bad habits. These habits in turn lead to negative thoughts listed above. Such emotions may or may not affect the person at whom these are directed, but these certainly harm the person himself, who persists in holding such emotions. Many people develop depression due to past disappointments. Anxiety is for uncertain future. It is scientifically proved that such emotional toxins disturb your peace, affect your white blood cells, reduce your immunity and make you prone to get various diseases.

Emotional toxins are very subtle sub-atomic vibrations, which affect our subtle body (variously called astral body, aura, vital body, pranic body etc). Such emotional contamination has been documented by the modern techniques of Kirlian Aura Photography, which has been done on thousands of patients. The detail discussion of such techniques is out of the scope for this book. In Indian Yoga science, existence of subtle invisible bodies, Panch-Kosha, is well explained. Emotional disturbances lead to disturbed sleep, faulty digestion, and impaired elimination of toxic wastes from the body and invite ill health. On the other side, positive healthy emotions like kindness, sympathy, truthfulness, non-violence, tolerance, unselfish love, forgiveness are very important to HELP YOURSELF.

It is hard to forget or forgive many incidences in the life. But there is no use to brood over and bear the grudges for such incidents. You cannot forget but you could perhaps forgive, for your own sake. This does not express weakness or running away from the situation. By all means, try to correct the situation if you can. Try to improve the other person, AFTER you have improved yourself. Do it out of love. Hate the crime, not the criminal. Uproot the criminal tendencies, from your own mind and also from the others whenever you can. Do it gently, with love, with real sympathy. I know it is a hard task. Many would call it as a weakness of character. We are here on this planet to learn, to improve and to experience the peace and happiness. This is process of self-training, self-improvement. Before we demand improvement in others, let us look within ourselves. See what we can do for our own Self.

Conclusion:
To summarize, the purpose of this chapter is not to confuse the reader more than he already might be. All the different causes, which might be affecting your health in general and making you more prone to get cancer, are listed. On the brighter side, staying away from such factors and avoiding these cancer-producing influences might give you better chance to prevent cancer. Although there is no guarantee that such things will prevent cancer all the time and in all the cases, healthy lifestyles and staying away from harmful habits will no doubt improve your health to a great extent.

CHAPTER 5

EARLY DIAGNOSIS

For dealing with any problem, accurate diagnosis is very important. If the diagnosis is accurate, then there is better chance of taking right steps. This chapter deals with some standard approaches and some novel diagnostic tools for very early detection of cancer. The mainstream medical specialists may not accept some of these novel diagnostic approaches. These are my personal observations and opinions. I do not claim that all these techniques are guaranteed to make correct diagnosis about the presence or the absence of cancer. Many techniques are still experimental and may not be available locally. This chapter is being written for the information of the reader and not to direct him/ her either for, or against, any particular technique. The book " Alternative Medicine Definitive Guide To Cancer" by Burton Goldberg, Future Medicine Publishing, Tiburon, California, has been a reference source for my current writings. Reader should consult his own doctor before opting for any particular tests.

Invisible Cancer:
Cancer like cells are circulating in body most of the time. These cells are effectively caught and destroyed by our healthy immune system. Hence it is much better to strengthen our immune system so that cancer cells, even if present in our body, will not grow and lead to cancer disease. Mere presence of few cancer like cells in the body is not clinically the cancer disease. Only when such cells establish, spread and grow unchallenged, cancer makes its foothold and then becomes a disease. These stages may take from few months to many years. In some patients, small microscopic cancer may remain unchanged for many years. A person may die naturally or due to some other disease at a mature age and only at autopsy such tumors are accidentally discovered. This is especially true in cancer of prostate, a disease of old age. Here the cancer could be looked at as a co-existing, unwanted companion tumor. Careful thoughts must be given to various natural

therapies for small microscopic tumors that are not causing any symptoms. Obviously, such tumors need a close watch under medical supervision. Heroic aggressive treatments are not necessary. We have to make sure that the treatment is not worse than the disease.

Cancer Check-ups:
Cancer check-ups, as conducted in various clinics and hospitals, usually involve clinical examination by a doctor in addition to routine blood tests and X-ray of chest. Additional tests are ordered by the doctor as per the specific complaints of the patient. These methods are helpful to some extent but are not 100% guarantee against cancer. These tests provide some sense of security. Sometimes, check-ups may lead to more testing in the persons, if cancer is suspected. As stated before, cancer is a disease of cells. A cell is a very small microscopic structure. When only few cells are affected in cancer, there may be very few symptoms and signs for the diagnosis of cancer. It is nearly impossible to diagnose cancer in very early stage at cellular level. Even in a cubic millimeter tumor, which is like a pinch-size tumor, there might be as many as 1 million (10 lacs) cancer cells. Unless the tumor becomes at least 2-3 millimeters in diameter, it cannot be seen on any X-rays or modern scanning methods such as CT scan or MR scan. Cytology or biopsy, which is the study of cells under microscope, is much more sensitive technique but it cannot be routinely practiced on wide scale on healthy people routinely. Furthermore, even if such a routine cytology/ biopsy/ X-ray/ Scan were performed and the reports were found to be normal, there would be no guarantee that the same test few months later would come normal. The currently invisible cancer may become visible within the next 6 months, after one year or at any later time. We have to consider these facts before we can understand about the early detection of cancer. The currently available laboratory tests have these obvious limitations. This does not mean that such tests should be avoided. These tests should be done for early detection in people who have got some reason to undergo such testing.

When a tumor or an ulcer becomes visible, biopsy is the most reliable test for cancer diagnosis. Before we go into this further, let us review some other tests, which might be useful in early detection of cancer. Cancer cells, unlike normal cells, sometimes cause immune activation through antigen-antibody reactions. Antigen could be any biological substance (virus, toxin, fungus, bacteria, parasite, protein molecule) that the body comes to regard as a foreigner not belonging to the body. In cancer, antigen is a small protein molecule on the surface of a cancer cell. This enemy is sensed by the immune system especially by lymphocytes, our white blood cells. These sensor cells go near the antigen and react with it to form what is known as an antibody. Antibody gets attached to antigen and thus destroys the antigen. Thus a disease-causing antigen is neutralized. If the production of antibodies is deficient or slow compared to production of antigens, the immune system cannot cope and the disease progresses. These antigens and antibodies, even if present in very small quantity, can be detected in the blood of the patient. Sometimes, cancer cells produce certain chemicals that are called tumor markers.

Few important tests are mentioned below for the information of the reader. It is strongly advised that the reader himself or herself should consult own doctors before considering any of these tests.

PAP Test:
A technique such as PAP smear, which examines secretions from vagina, is advocated for screening of cancer of uterus in women. The PAP test would be able to detect very early changes in the cells appearing suspicious. However, for majority of solid tumors, which are hidden deep within the body, needle cytology or biopsies are the only methods for accurate diagnosis. Obviously, these techniques, which need attending a specialized medical clinic, and which might involve a cost to the patient, would not be feasible for screening of cancer in majority of the population. PAP test is also performed for oral cancer, esophageal cancer and gastric cancer, where secretions from the tumor can be collected on a swab.

PSA:

PSA is a test used for detection of cancer of prostate. PSA stands for Prostate-Specific-Antigen. This is a blood test. Raised PSA is suspicious for cancer of prostate. PSA is marginally raised even in non-cancerous enlarged prostate or in infection of prostate. The test has some false positive and false negative results. It has to be considered together with medical examination by a physician. PSA testing is more important to monitor the progress of the patient of prostate cancer. The test is available in all the modern laboratories, although it is somewhat expensive.

AMAS:
This test is not readily available even in developed countries. The test claims to diagnose most of the cancers in early stage, when there are no other signs to suggest cancer. This test was developed by a Harvard trained physician, Dr. Sam Bogoch in 1990s after 20 years work in laboratory. AMAS stands for "Anti-Malignin-Antibody-Screen". It assumes that all the cancer cells have a common surface antigen on the cancer cell wall. This antigen produces a common antibody in most of the cancers. The antibody level is measured in AMAS. If raised, there is a high probability of some type of cancer in the body. The physician then can order more specific tests for cancer location. When the cancer tumor is obvious, this test is not necessary. This test is available through Dr. Bogoch's Oncolab at 36 The Fenway, Boston, MA 02215. (USA phone: 1-800-922-8387). The test is expensive and not easy to order from abroad.

Tumor Markers:
Many cancer growths secrete certain chemicals, which are called tumor markers. CEA, CA-15, CA-125, Beta- HCG, Alfa-feto- proteins are names of some of such tests for tumor markers. These tests are usually employed after the diagnosis of cancer to see the extent of cancer and to monitor the progress of cancer. These are not routinely used for early detection of cancer. Besides these common tumor markers, many other tumor marker tests are being developed. In breast cancer, ER (estrogen receptor) and PR (progesterone receptor) tests serve important role in planning the treatment of the patient.

Mammography:
This is a test with special X-Ray technique to highlight the internal structure of the breast. The most basic way to detect breast tumor is by self- examination or by the examination done by a doctor. Majority of the breast lumps are benign. Only a small proportion is cancerous. Mammography may serve some purpose for women at high risk for developing breast cancer. The mammography is somewhat painful and involves use of X-rays, which in turn could have some minimal hazards. Although being promoted as routine screening test for large sections of population, the cost-benefit ratio of this technique is controversial. Besides being controversial, recommendation for routine periodic mammography in all women above say 40 years of age could lead to anxiety and cancer-panic. Screening with mammography in every woman might not be cost effective and may be counter-productive. There is a suggestion that mammography may detect a large number of slow growing tumors which may not be highly malignant. Such tumors, although cancerous under microscope, might not lead to the usual aggressive breast cancer, which takes the toll of the patient in a short time. Such slow growing tumors might need only periodic observation rather than any prompt surgery, chemotherapy, radiotherapy etc.

According to Dr. David Plotkin, M.D. (Plotkin, D., "Good News and Bad News about Breast Cancer." The Atlantic Monthly, -June 1996, page 82), "Mammography is only leading physicians to diagnose an ever-larger number of harmless breast tumors. Patients who otherwise would never have known they have a tumor may needlessly suffer through the unique pain, anxiety, disfigurement and expense associated with modern medicine and cancer." While a mammogram may accurately indicate a tumor, it can not in itself tell what time it will take to double its own size. Many slow cancers have tumor doubling times more than 15 to 20 years. A 1 cm small tumor detected in a 60 year old woman may perhaps become 2 cm large, without causing any trouble at all, when the women reaches 80 years of age. In effect, the woman co-exists with her slow cancer without the need for any toxic chemotherapy, radiation or surgery. Of course the woman should make her own choice about whether she needs such tests and what further management she would be prepared to undergo, with advice from an open minded doctor. This is the age of information and the patients should be given various options, explaining merits and demerits of each line of treatment. Each person should be able to decide his / her own options especially in a disease like cancer, where the modern treatments cannot guarantee any cures.

Hemoccult Test:
Testing stools for trace of blood is a simple but an important test. Tumors in colon and rectum usually bleed and the blood passes in the stool. If the amount of the blood is large, a person can notice the bleeding for himself. However, early cancer in colon may pass only very small amount of blood, which cannot be seen by eyes. The test for occult blood in the stool can detect small traces of blood. This test could be done as an initial screening in patients with high risk of colon cancer.

Endoscopy:
Passing special fiber-optic tubes with lights and camera to study various cavities of body is known as Endoscopy- inner viewing. Routine use of these tests for mass screening is not feasible. These tests serve very useful purpose for early detection in the patients at risk of cancer. Laryngoscopy, Bronchoscopy, Gastroscopy, Colonoscopy, Proctoscopy, Peritonoscopy are some names of the endoscopies related to different areas of body.

Darkfield Microscopy:
Since the use of standard microscope has failed to detect any signs of germs in cancer tissue, it was believed until recently that blood contained no living organism that could contribute to cancer. Standard microscopy and even electron microscopy, due to it's staining and preparations, lead to death of any living matter on the slides. This makes any observations about small living particles in the cells impossible. Only well recognized forms of dead bacteria, viruses and fungi could be identified by such techniques. Darkfield microscopy,

which is the examination of live blood smear without staining under reflected light in a dark field, has been supplying compelling evidence about existence of such live particles, which may be responsible in cancer causation. Experienced doctors can detect abnormal forms of blood cells together with living motile particles called protits and somatids. Conversion of these protits and somatids to aggressive forms is associated with cancer. Besides cancer, darkfield microscopy is useful in detection of various other chronic and acute diseases. This technique is not readily available in common laboratories or even in modern hospitals. A French Canadian scientist Gaston Naessens, Prof. Günter Enderlein from Germany and Dr Virginia Livingston Wheeler from USA are few scientists who have done pioneering research in this field. Darkfield microscopy, although easy to learn for health practitioners, is not commonly available.

Biological Terrain Assessment:
This is a phrase used to describe the internal biochemical conditions, general health and activity at cellular level. Body maintains precise pH, which is a measure of acidity/ alkalinity of various tissues and fluids in the body. Blood is kept at a pH of 7.34 to 7.4. Foods used for life process create acidity or alkalinity in the body. Metabolism of foods is a process of Oxidation-Reduction. To liberate energy from foods we eat, the process of oxidation-reduction is being continuously used in all the cells. Certain foods can lead to creation of excessive oxidative radicals, which are called free radicals or oxidative stress. These free radicals are highly reactive and could cause many harmful chemical reactions in cells. Such reactions lead to cellular toxicity, improper cellular function and to ill health. Tissues conduct electricity for various biological functions. This conductivity has to be kept at an optimal level for good health. Measurement of pH, oxidative stress and electrical conductivity of certain tissues is known as assessment of Biological Terrain. There are various instruments and laboratory tests developed to assess the biochemical activities of the body and to assess tissue toxicity. These tests also suggest ways to correct any abnormal findings, mostly with diet and nutritional products. BTA, CBC, Maverick Test, Pantox Profile, Metamatrix Toxmet Screen are names of some of the patented

laboratory tests being used in USA for such screening tests. Other tests assess the tumor antigens, cell sub-populations and lymphocyte size to predict cancerous trends. Interested reader may refer to the book "Alternative Medicine Definitive Guide to Cancer" by Burton Goldberg.

X-Rays:
Since the discovery of X-Rays by Wilhelm Roentgen of Germany in 1895, X-rays became an important part of the modern medical science. With X-rays, it was possible to see and photograph internal organs of body! X-rays were used for diagnosis and treatment of countless medical conditions. In an X-ray tube, invisible rays are produced when very high voltage electrical current is applied. These rays can go through the body and take a picture of internal structures; much like a camera takes pictures of the outside world. With use of various contrast media, the x-ray machines can take precise pictures of the internal organs like stomach, kidneys, gall bladder, blood vessels, heart, lungs, brain etc. This is the science of radiology.

Scans:
In the past few decades, very sophisticated techniques were developed to take pictures of internal organs. CT Scan machines (Computed Tomography) use a large number of simultaneous X-ray beams penetrating through body. Computer then develops a composite radiographic picture of a particular slice of any body part. Nuclear medicine has various techniques to see internal organs concentrating the radioactive isotopes injected into the body. These are called isotope scans. Isotope scans for bone, liver, brain and other organs are being used for medical diagnosis. MR (Magnetic Resonance) scan, a recent addition, use strong magnetic pulses to cause transient changes in the orientation of water molecules, which are present in every cell and tissue. By changing patterns of such water molecules (specifically the protons of the hydrogen atoms in water molecule), internal organs become visible on Magnetic Resonance (MR) scan. Ultrasound scans, called sonography, use high frequency sound waves to traverse through body parts and take pictures of internal organs. PET scan and SPECT

scans are names of some other rarely used scanning techniques for imaging of internal organs. As a rule, these scans will see any tumor only when it is at least a few millimeters in size. As stated earlier, a cubic millimeter of tumor might contain about 1 million cancer cells! These scans cannot see individual cancer cells. X-rays and scans can see small tumors, but at this stage cancer cells have already established a foothold in the body. Again, these tests will point out to small tumors but would be unable to tell if it is a cancer or some other type of shadow. Compared to these imaging x-rays and scans, the tests for tumor markers and tumor antigens are much more precise and helpful for early detection of cancer. X-rays and nuclear radiations used for medical diagnosis and medical treatment are known to cause cancer in exposed people. Hence the use of X-rays and other radiations has to be done with great caution.

Biopsy:
Biopsy is the Mother of All Tests for Cancer. Without biopsy, cancer diagnosis is not complete. In biopsy, a small portion of tumor is removed and seen under microscope. An experienced pathologist can very easily see the signs of cancer in the slide under microscope. Cancer cell is larger, irregular and has darkly staining large nucleus within cell. Signs of disorder, invasion and encroachment are abundant. Cancer can be classified to exact type as per the microscopic appearance. Carcinoma is name given to malignancy arising from linings of the internal organs or skin surface. Squamous cell carcinoma arises from the mucous lining or skin surface. Adeno-carcinoma arises from the lining of glandular tissue such as stomach, colon, breast etc. Carcinoma could be of high grade or low grade. Higher the grade, more aggressive and dangerous the spread of cancer. Sarcoma is term used for malignant tumors arising from connective tissues such as bones, fats, muscles, cartilage etc, which are not communicating with outer surfaces or with inner cavities in the body. Leukemia is name used for cancer of blood, which is the liquid of life constantly on the move through veins and arteries. Initially, leukemia does not form any localized solid tumors, although when advanced, secondary tumors are seen in various parts of body. Lymphoma is the term used for tumors originating in lymph

nodes and organs connected with the lymphatic system of body. Myeloma is a special type of tumor primarily starting in bone marrow without involving any other organs, at least in the beginning.

FNAC, Needle Biopsy, Punch Biopsy, Excision Biopsy, Incision Biopsy, Endoscopic Biopsy are various terms used to describe different techniques of biopsy. FNAC stands for Fine Needle Aspiration Cytology. With a very thin needle, a drop is aspirated from the suspected tumor area. Some tumor cells come in the drop, which can be studied under microscope. Needle biopsy tries to remove a little larger length of tumor tissue, which is easier to study and which can provide more precise diagnosis. Punch biopsy uses even larger forceps to punch out a part of tumor.

When the tumor is large, it is incised and only a part of tumor is removed for study. This is called incision biopsy as opposed to excision biopsy where the whole tumor is removed in one piece for pathological study. Biopsy is usually done before any major surgical operation to confirm the diagnosis of cancer and to see the exact type of cancer. This information helps a great deal to plan the operation. Before planning major operation, in addition to the biopsy, x-rays, scans and blood tests are performed to rule out the spread of cancer to other organs. If cancer is widespread, major operations are of little use to control the cancer.

After the biopsy the chunk of tumor is treated with certain chemicals and then embedded in a paraffin wax to make a small paraffin block. Very thin sections of such blocks can be sliced, put on glass slides and made ready for examination under microscope. An expert pathologist can study such slides and give his/ her opinion about cancer. After a major operation to remove the cancer, the entire tumor together with surrounding tissue is sent to the surgical pathologist for detailed examination of the whole specimen. Lymph nodes, small glands around the tumor, are also removed to see if the tumor cells have already gone into these areas. The lymph nodes are like police stations, which are supposed to screen the flow of the lymph and arrest any unwanted cells, germs or toxins. When the tumor is aggressive, it goes through the lymph nodes and spreads in distant areas of the body. This is then called the advanced stage of tumor. Sometimes, tumor cells, bypassing lymph nodes, travel through blood circulation and land in distant organs. This is called distant metastasis. When the cancer tumor spreads to lymph nodes, it is called as 2nd or 3rd stage. When the distant organs show metastasis of cancer, it is very advanced 4th stage.

Conclusion:

In summary, cancer diagnosis is difficult in very early stage. The symptoms are vague and can simulate many other disease conditions. Initially, doctors usually may not order all the tests to rule out all the types of cancer. Many times this intensive medical testing is not feasible. Furthermore, patients are also reluctant for so many tests because of economical difficulties, psychological fear and inconvenience of such medical tests. Normal tests at any particular time do not guarantee that the patient will never have cancer. Since the cancer cells are very small and since these cells grow slowly, mostly unnoticed by our immune system, cancer can become visible at any later date. Therefore, such tests for cancer detection should be undertaken with understanding of their scope and limitations.

CHAPTER 6

TREATMENT OF CANCER, THE CORE

Diagnosis of cancer is the initial big shock to the patient and the relatives. There is sudden despair, fear and panic in the family. The thoughts of painful treatments, uncertain outcome, exorbitant expenses and general anxiety dominate the family members. The first question invariably is " Can Cancer Be Cured?" The answer is difficult. It is not easy to answer this question with a simple Yes or No! There are thousands and thousands examples of cancer survivors, even from terminal stage! There are examples of many so called "spontaneous cures". Patients, who were given " Only few months to live" by their medical doctors, have beaten the "Judgment". To the amazement of the friend's bewilderment of medical scientists, these patients are around for 5, 10, 15, 20 years or even longer after the D-Day! Whatever the statistics predict, a patient is either alive or dead, 100%. They're no such thing as 70 % survival rate or 80% mortality rate for an individual patient. The patient wants to get cured, by whatever means possible.

In following chapters, I will describe various conventional and not so conventional cancer treatments. I am trying to outline the overall strategy for dealing with cancer. I do not claim that any of these treatments will guarantee cure from cancer. The information is given for the readers. Any particular line of treatment mentioned here should be undertaken under the advice of your own doctor and under proper supervision. In general, to be successful, one should start with the attitude " Cancer Can Be Cured!"

In a book called "Remarkable Recovery" published by Institute of Noetic Science, hundreds and hundreds of cases of victory over cancer, which was pronounced incurable by orthodox medicine, have been given. All these patients had faith and positive attitude, which enabled them to fight cancer. Patients followed various novel methods to conquer their cancer, but the common factor was a positive attitude and lifestyle changes to healthier way of life. Most of such conquest could not be explained by the modern medicine and were termed as spontaneous cures!

Recently, there has been vigorous interest in scientific studies about the benefits of complementary cancer treatments and holistic approach. Several scientific medical studies document the benefits of complementary medical therapies. Following are just a few examples of such trials.

1. In a study conducted at University of California, LA, in Melanoma, a deadly skin cancer, psychological support therapy to the patients for 1.5 hours weekly for 6 weeks reduced the recurrence rates and increased the survival 300%.
2. In a Hawaii study on 675 patients of lung cancer, it was observed that the group, which had highest vegetable intake, had double the survival rates compared to the group, which had lowest vegetable intake.
3. A randomized study in Detroit on cancer of prostate patients observed that 15 mg of lycopenes (found in red tomatoes) given daily for 3 weeks before the operation caused partial shrinkage of the prostate cancer and reduced PSA level.
4. Patients under chemotherapy receiving antioxidants and micronutrients therapy had 30% fewer damage to the bone marrow cells. Micronutrients are special vitamins, minerals and supplements found to promote health.
5. Breast cancer patients on chemotherapy, who were given high doses of Vitamin A, had nearly double the improvement rates.
6. In a recent paper in New England Journal of Medicine, drinking green tea has been shown to reduce the risk of cancer of bladder.
7. Essential fatty acids in fish oil together with natural vitamin E given to advance stage cancer patients has shown to triple the estimated survival periods.

There are countless papers and publications in recent years on treatment of cancer and other chronic diseases with the help of complementary medical treatments.

It is obvious that to get better results, the treatment strategy for cancer should be much more than only to consider standard approaches of surgery, radiation therapy and chemotherapy. Basically, one has to consider the cancer treatment in three parts.

1. FUNDAMENTAL CORE: Attend to internal and external microenvironment of the individual. Resolve any emotional conflicts. Create positive attitude.
2. FOUNDATION: Attend to lifestyles, habits, nutrition, exercise, relaxation, and detoxification regimens.
3. THERAPY: Decide upon surgery, radiation therapy, chemotherapy, immunotherapy, herbal therapy, and other complementary therapies such as Ayurved, Acupuncture, Homeopathy and many others.

All the above points should be considered simultaneously or possibly even before definitive standard treatments like surgery, radiation therapy and chemotherapy. As we all are aware, these conventional treatments are directed only against the cancer tumor and give little attention to the person who has cancer. Radiation and chemotherapy, although effective in destroying cancer cells, usually cause lot of reactions and interfere with the natural immunity of the body. Normal tissues and normal cells also suffer significant damage during these attacks on cancer cells. Hence, to enable normal tissues to survive and fight against cancer, attention to the core and to the foundation is very important. This focus would certainly improve the results of any current cancer treatments and would help to control the cancer disease better.

THE CORE

First we have to look in to the "core" of the patient, which consists of his/ her personality, emotions, belief systems and "Will to Live".

Bhagavad-Gita says, " Mind is the prime cause for human liberation as well as the bondage". This also applies to worldly affairs such as health, happiness, and success. Wise people all over the world, throughout all the ages, understood the power of mind over matter. One has to ask certain questions to oneself to analyze own mind. If the person is unable to do it himself, others should help him do so. Close relatives, friends, social workers, psychologists and even doctors should attend to this aspect. The core is all-important for health and happiness as well as for disease and misery. The questions to be asked are:

1. Am I happy about myself and for my life so far?
2. Do I feel desperate or disappointed about my life?
3. Do I feel hopeless about the future?
4. Do I want to live? Do I wish to get better?
5. Do I blame others for my suffering?
6. Do I feel guilty about important events in my life?
7. Am I depressed about the past events?
8. Am I anxious about the future?
9. What are my fears?
10. Do I feel isolated and lonely?
11. What are my conflicts?
12. Am I in the habit of "proving my worth" to others?

I am fully aware that very few men and women would be able to give healthy answers to these questions. One has to be open to analyze and accept, at least for himself / herself, the emotional problems one is facing. Many patients subconsciously suppress despair, grief, disappointments, guilt, insults, fears etc. Life is a trial, and usually a hard one. It is mixture of pleasures and pains. Mostly, pains outweigh the pleasures. When we are unable to express our hurts, things gather steam internally and sooner or later these manifest as health problems. Persons who can find a vent to these pressures have a better chance of recovery than those who suffer silently! Quiet desperation is root cause for various health problems. Only one thing is perfectly clear that no one is perfect in this world. As Elisabeth Kubler-Ross said, cultivate the attitude " I am not OK, You are not OK, but that is OK". Try to bring your hurts, guilt, doubts, and insecurities in open with family and friends. Most of the times, nothing could be done to remedy the events, which have caused emotional trauma. Bringing them in open could be a major treatment for such suffering. Many persons would not even be aware about their emotional suppressions. They are resigned to the suffering and may subconsciously wish to find a way out. Cancer is such an escape for some of us. If a person, with the help of supportive family and friends, is able to reverse these negative trends, chances of beating the cancer are markedly improved. Modern medical doctors are trained to be body mechanics. In medical school, we are led to believe that everything could be "fixed" from external efforts. Patient need not participate in this fight over the disease. Patient just has to follow "doctor's orders". Doctors know the best. Modern medicine, reluctant to acknowledge the power of mind, has almost discounted presence of mind in treatment protocols. Once a disease label is decided, each patient with that condition gets the same treatment. Focus is on treating cancer tumor rather than treating a person who has cancer! We doctors are taught to prolong the life, at any cost. We try to keep a terminal patient, with tubes in all the body openings and needles in veins, alive as long as possible. That is called "success". Death is considered a "failure". Curiously, everybody seems to eventually die. As Dr. Bernie Siegel said "Death is not the issue. Life is. Death is not a failure. Not to take the challenge of life is." Hence there is a lot of work to be done at "core" level, simultaneously with the attack on cancer tumor. Earlier in the chapter of "Causes of Cancer", we have seen how mind can promote as well as prevent cancer.

Mind-Body Medicine:
How to do this? Core treatment is most difficult but potentially most rewarding type of therapy. The usual tranquilizers, sedatives and sleeping pills cannot correct the root cause. Usually, such pills only mask the mental symptoms and may produce side effects like drowsiness, disorientation, heavy headedness, clouding of alertness etc. Hence the speciality of Mind-Body Medicine is now being looked upon with new hope.

The aim of Mind-body medicine is to help the patient to help himself. Here, the patient has to participate himself in own healing. A lot of help is needed from family, friends and professionals. If successful, this would not only help reduce cancer tumor but could make one a happy and healthy person. The motto of Mind-Body medicine is to " Empower mind to help body heal". A patient has to develop positive attitude. He should take the challenge and look at cancer as a milestone to find new meaning to life, to be a better person, to be at peace with himself and with others. This is the time to take stock of what baggage is stored in the subconscious. It is the time to seek new directions, proclaim new affirmations, to expand one's perspective of life. Techniques of Mind-Body medicine can be considered as follows:

1. Nurturing spiritual beliefs based upon natural laws (Dharma, Religious truths)
2. Meditation, Mental concentration with japa, raja-yoga, bhakti-yoga, etc
3. Pranayama and other breathing practices to purify mind and body.
4. Auto-suggestions
5. Biofeedback
6. Visualization
7. Hypnosis
8. Spiritual Healing, Reiki, Therapeutic Touch, Prayers,

Spiritual Belief Systems:

Although banished from the world by the "science", the existence of higher power (call it God if you will), guiding the evolution of the universe cannot be denied by a thinking mind. For our human evolution from ego-centric mind to super-mind, we need to assume validity of certain universal truths perceived by our own metaphysical scientists that are saints, rishis, seers, prophets who have actually experienced these truths. Our logical mind is quick to trust the words of Prof. XYZ or Doctor ABC in mundane matters. However our little ego would not accept the existence of some invisible superior principle like God. We deny the universal super-ego fearing subjugation of our little personal ego to higher ego. Ego resists extinction. That is the reason why all of us fear death, which we think as "The End". Ego, by divine instinct, is immortal. Ego cannot tolerate the idea of it's own destruction. Body is identified with ego. We want to pamper, care, comfort, adorn, adore and love our own bodies by whatever means possible. We seek pleasure and hate pain. Disease means suffering. All the efforts are made to remove this suffering of body-mind-ego complex. Experiments with natural truths are like scientific experiments conducted in a laboratory. Only here, the body is your tool, your mind is the student and the world is your laboratory. You have to assume certain hypotheses to start the experiment of the life- time. Even for a degree in physics, maths, medicine etc, you have to pursue the required course of studies for many years and pass the exam. In spiritual matters, premature denial of natural truths by dry logic, without doing adequate experiments in a proper manner (read it as " Saadhana"), cannot qualify you for graduation! You might have to return, again and again, to this world to earn your degree of liberation. There are no short cuts.

On practical side, a person has to discover self-love. When born, a baby is full of contentment and love. As long as the basic physical needs of hunger, sleep and security are taken care of, the baby is happy. The baby is not worried about the bank balance or job security. The baby soon catches up with the manners of the world. Likes and dislikes are learnt. Feelings of love or rejection and insecurity are created. The child then tries to win the love of parents. Upbringing of a child in a healthy manner is most important for the future health and happiness of the child. Very few grown-ups truly love themselves, as they are. There are endless lines of cosmetics and designer clothes to help us look better than we are. I apologize for this sermon, but I wish only to peel off the outer layers from the inner core so that we could focus our attention on the reality within. Belief in divine justice and divine grace certainly helps us to face the trials of life successfully. Patients who are happy and who love themselves suffer much less health problems and do recover faster if they develop any diseases. This also is true for a disease like cancer. The first principle therefore is " Never give up hope". You can make a miracle happen. As David Ben-Gurien once said " Anyone who does not believe in miracles is not a realist".

Meditation, Yoga and Pranayama:

Meditation has been described in great details in scriptures and various books on yoga, philosophy, religions and health sciences. Various techniques are given. Meditation is called by various names such as relaxation response (coined by Dr. Herbert Benson of Harvard), dipping in core, uniting with self, searching the ego, Quest for Self etc. All these techniques try to remove the block in the way of your conscious mind to reach your inner self, which is the real storehouse of universal energy. If you are successful in communicating with your inner self, all this benign energy is yours to use. This is a long process requiring commitment, faith and regularity of practice. Regular meditation is beneficial, not only for cancer patients, but also for all those who wish to be happy, healthy and prosperous. Yoga is union of your little self with the Universal Self. Various paths such as bhakti-yoga (devotion), japa-yoga (repetition of Name or Word), karma-yoga (selfless deeds), gyan-yoga (reaching the truth with discrimination), hatha-yoga, raja-yoga ultimately lead to the same goal. Pranayama, control of breath, is a technique described in yoga texts. Various breathing techniques are described that can lead to sublimation of negative thoughts, purification from thought pollutions, mental concentration, good health and ultimately samadhi. Samadhi is your union with your inner core. It is the supreme experience of infinite bliss, power and peace. Meditation, yoga and pranayama should be learnt under proper guru and should be practiced regularly for success.

Mudra & Aasana:

Mudra and aasana are of special help in meditation and pranayama. Aasana, specific postures prescribed in Yoga texts, are a great help for meditation and mental concentration. Different aasana have been shown to improve the functions of different internal organs. Mudra is a specific posture of the fingers of hands held during meditation and pranayama. Subtle energy channels carrying prana, vital energy, run through all the parts of our body. In yoga texts, these are described as nadis. In Chinese acupuncture, these channels are called meridians. At the tips of the fingers, subtle energy channels are very active. Various spots on fingertips are connected to various internal organs by means of nadis or meridians. Joining two or more fingertips in certain fashion creates a mudra. Such mudra can help circulate the prana, the vital energy, through various internal organs of the body. Many mudras, e.g. gyan-mudra, dhyan-mudra, linga-mudra, prana-mudra, vayu-mudra, prithvi-mudra etc are described with their individual health benefits. In a recent clinical study on carpel tunnel syndrome, it was shown that mudra therapy produced significant improvement in pain in hands and wrists without operation. Carpel tunnel syndrome is due to pressure on the muscles and nerves at the wrists, for which an operation to open the wrist space is undertaken.

Autosuggestions and Affirmations:

These are practical daily routines to communicate with your subconscious mind to bring about many benefits. As stated by Louise Hay in her book Heal Your Body, cancer is usually caused by deep hurt, longstanding resentments, unresolved grief eating away at the self, carrying hatred, hopelessness, unresolved despair. Affirmation is speaking to your own subconscious mind directing it to correct a mental block. Affirmations are done daily as you wake up and also just before you go to bed every day. You repeat a sentence with full trust that required benefit is already happening. There are countless examples of changes in attitudes and healing of so many persons. For cancer, Louise Hays suggests following affirmation: *" I lovingly forgive and release all of the past. I choose to fill my world with joy. I love and approve myself."* She also gives a list of negative mental attitudes and corrective affirmations for various other diseases. Interested reader may refer to her book "Heal Your Body" published in USA by Hay House, Inc., California.

Autosuggestions have similar effects. Suggestions for what you wish to happen should be quietly spoken to your own mind at the time of waking and just before bedtime. These are the periods when sleeping and waking states are interchanging. This is the moment when subconscious mind is especially receptive to any suggestion from the conscious mind. Infants and small children, who are unable to make affirmations themselves, could be helped by mother or father. A parent can whisper the affirmation in the ear of the child at the right moment, regularly. Although consciously unable to understand the affirmation, the child will have subconscious impressions of the affirmation to bring about the required benefits. Autosuggestions can also be passively transmitted to a patient in coma by relatives and friends. The whole idea of these affirmations, meditations, yoga etc is to uncover the fountain of love and energy, which has been hidden due to the "teachings of the world".

Biofeedback:
Biofeedback means sending voluntary signals to internal organs to change their function. There are voluntary muscles, like those of hands, feet, voice box, back etc whose actions are under our conscious control. We can start or stop such actions at will. There are involuntary muscles like those of heart, stomach, intestines, inner glands, which do their work automatically. These are not under our conscious control. These activities are under control of autonomic nervous system. Technique of serial contraction and relaxation of voluntary muscles can indirectly control the action of the autonomic nervous system. This is the basis of biofeedback. In the west, Edmond Jacobson first described in 1908 the technique of progressive muscular relaxation leading to various internal changes in the autonomic nervous system. This became the basis for biofeedback therapy. In India under British Rule, there are numerous recorded testimonials about some yogis voluntarily stopping heartbeats or suspending respiration for long time. These yogis could later bring the suspended functions back to normal. This could be called oriental style of biofeedback!

A person can be taught to contract and relax groups of muscles, which in turn would reduce the blood pressure, prevent attack of migraine etc by an effect on autonomic nervous system function. The desired effect can be linked with an audio-visual signal the patient can see. For example, a person with high blood pressure starts this muscular relaxation exercise. At the desired number, say 120 mm systolic blood pressure, a bell would ring announcing the patient has been successful in bringing down his own blood pressure at the desired level. Here the patient feels in control of the situation since he is rewarded with audio-visual signal of his own success. Similar techniques have been developed for many other conditions. Biofeedback is more acceptable technique for a scientifically oriented inquisitive person. He can see the rewards of his own efforts on a machine! There is no need for imagination. Patients can be conditioned for certain predictable response during the biofeedback therapy. I remember Dr. Datey, a well-known senior cardiologist in Bombay, successfully treating patients of high blood pressure in 1960s with shavasana, a technique similar to biofeedback. I am not sure how biofeedback might be helpful in cancer treatments. Perhaps by reducing stress and physical pains, it might provide the patient some feeling of being in control.

Visualization & Imagery:
Here a patient is taught to visualize with his mental eye, sequences of healthy scenes. With his mind, he sees that he is breathing pure air, smelling fragrance of fresh flowers, he is sitting near a beautiful riverbank and listening to mystic sounds of running water, or he is at the top of a mountain witnessing the splendors of the rising sun. He visualizes being bathed by healthy rays from the morning sun. Various health-promoting scenes are depicted by the patient in his mind's eye. He is told to actually believe that he is physically experiencing all these goodies of the nature. After that he is told to turn is attention to the happenings within his body. He then visualizes tuning up the functions of various internal organs to optimal levels, and then he visualizes the strengthening of his immune system, white blood cells, macrophages, and natural killer cells. Then he visualizes that this white blood cells immune force is attacking his black cancer cells and destroying them one by one. Repeated and regular visualization of such mental images has actually shown to improve immunity and destroy cancer cells.

To be successful, all the mind-body techniques described so far need a high level of self-motivation, persistence and positive efforts on the part of the patient.

Hypnosis:

Hypnosis is a state of attentive and focused concentration. Hypnotherapist can induce a trance and slowly take a patient into deeper levels of subconscious mind. The subject goes into a trance but is partly aware of the surroundings. It is not like a sleep where a person is not aware of anything. In hypnotic trance, a person is highly responsive to the commands of the therapist. Therapist then issues some commands and the body usually follows the instructions. Some persons are more easily hypnotized than others. Undoubtedly, personality of individual is important in being "hypnotized". We did conduct some experiments with hypnosis on some cancer patients in early 1990s in Bombay. We observed that hypnosis offered good pain relief and relaxation in some cancer patients. Whether it can destroy cancer cells, I am not sure. It might be complementary treatment in certain patients for general improvement.

Spiritual Healing, Prayers etc:

Here a therapist, who sincerely wishes to help a patient, acts as a channel for the universal energy. Spiritual healers can usually detect disturbances in the invisible aura around visible physical body. Yoga science has described 4 subtle bodies as sheaths around the visible physical body. These five sheaths are called panch kosha. These are 1. Physical 2. Vital-pranic, 3. Mental: Manomaya, 4. Intelligence: Vigyanamaya and lastly 5.Innermost Causal: Anandamaya kosha. Some spiritual healers and yogis claim that they can actually see these different sheaths surrounding the body. Aura is a bright colorful sheath of invisible light around all living beings. In disease, aura shows local changes of dull black-brown colors, corresponding to diseased organs. An experienced aura reader can detect various disturbances leading to different diseases. Such healers are able to "clean" or "clear" the defects in the aura somewhat similar to cleaning a dirty house, inside and out! There are testimonials of patients undergoing such spiritual healing feeling highly improved soon after such healing sessions. However, this might not have a long lasting health benefit unless the patient decides to keep his "house" clean by attending to periodic health maintenance. A house-cleaner can clean your house during his session but if you persist making your house (body) dirty by faulty lifestyles, the cleaning effect would not last forever.

Dr. Geoffery Morell, a spiritual healer from Washington, DC, frequently visits our centers in Mumbai and Pune to give healing sessions to patients here. I have personally witnessed his ability to feel the defects in aura and to accurately locate the places of tumors in many patients. Several patients have reported benefits from such healing sessions. For cancer, spiritual healing sessions could be used as a supplementary therapy to other specific treatments.

Reiki & Therapeutic Touch
Reiki is based on inviting the universal energy (Rei + Ki) to a patient through the hands of a reiki master. The technique of reiki sessions is slightly different from that of spiritual healing. An initiated reiki master can project various power transmitting symbols to the patient. Healing energy is thus transmitted from cosmic power to the patient, the therapist being only a channel. Reiki is supposed to have its own will and intelligence to effect a healing. Reiki was discovered by a Japanese Christian missionary, Dr. Usui, in the early part of 20th century. As per some reports, the art of reiki originated in India with Buddhist monks. Buddhist monks took this art to Tibet and other eastern nations later on, while it was forgotten in India. Now there is renewed interest in reiki all over the world. There are numerous reiki practitioners in India and in various nations around the world. Logical western mind, so far reluctant to admit anything that is not proved in a laboratory, is slowly coming to try these alternative mind-body techniques on increasing scale. A patient may use reiki as a complementary treatment to support his mainline cancer treatments. On its own, I doubt if reiki can destroy cancer tumor in an average patient. Therapeutic touch is based on similar principle and has similar scope and limitations. This can be learnt by any well-meaning person who sincerely wants to heal patients.

There are courses and books, which would help reader to know more about these techniques.

Prayers:
Prayers to mortal humans may not work but sincere prayers to higher truths, call it God if you will, certainly have effect on psyche of the recipients, for whom the prayers is done. It has been documented, time and again, that prayers do work. In all religious rituals, prayers occupy an important place. The validity of such spiritual techniques is beyond the understanding current science. However, what were once considered as unscientific blind beliefs were proved to be scientific facts later on when science advanced. Till 16th century in Europe, the earth was considered as stationary and at the center of the universe. In early 17th century, Galileo, who tried to say earth went round the sun, was persecuted. Now we know the facts. As the science progresses, some currently held scientific facts might have to be discarded later on. Blind science is as bad as blind faith.

Strive For A Goal:
Feelings of hopelessness, despair, rejection, loneliness, low self esteem cause depression and many other health problems. Such patients should be encouraged to find something in life worth living for. As per individual liking and capacity, a person can fix up some goal in his/ her mind. Striving for such a goal is one of the best treatments to uplift the spirit and come out of the negative mental blocks. A goal should be something concrete, material objective. Abstract objectives " I wish to be happy", "I want to achieve Nirvana" or "I want to find peace" cannot be considered as material goals. A mind needs a material goal to overcome physical illness. Pursuing a material goal within a fixed time frame can invigorate the body, mind and spirit.

Homeopathy as Mind-Body Medicine:
Homeopathy, a peculiar alternative medical science discovered by Samuel Hahnemann in Germany in 18th century, is not basically a mind-body technique. However, I have personally witnessed many amazing instances where homeopathy has been very helpful in dealing with

mental delusions, fears, and deep-seated mental wounds. It is said that one cannot change own nature. I can say that homeopathy can change negative mental reactions and unhealthy attitudes to a great extent. I find homeopathy especially helpful in dealing with psychosomatic illnesses, which result from mental stress. Flower remedies by Bach is another variation of homeopathy, which has been found helpful in dealing with health problems related to fright, fear, anxiety, grief, insecurity, panic, anger, depression etc. I will write about my personal experiences in this matter later in the chapter of "Psychology of Cancer". I would suggest that a patient could be helped by an experienced homeopathic practitioner if he / she has a lot of emotional problems and mood changes. Homeopathy can play a complementary role in overall cancer care.

Conclusion:

A revolution is going on to explore mind's power over the matter. Mind is the basic factor in causing as well as healing most of the sufferings. Various mind-body techniques are being developed and tried to see if such things can give better health prospects to the people. The revolution is going on especially because allopathic medicine, although efficient in dealing with emergency and acute diseases, has proved to be unsatisfactory in control of chronic diseases. In spite of more advances, more hospitals and more doctors, health care seems to be getting more complicated and less effective for the masses. The progress of the science in general, and medicine in particular, is technology oriented. Many times, practical applications of such discoveries are driven by commercial interests. People all over the world are looking for safer, gentle, natural, affordable and effective ways to deal with their health care. The model of mechanic doctor, able to fix everything, in the machine called body is changing. Patients need to be equal partners in their own health care. After all it is your body, which is suffering and you deserve to look for safe, gentle, natural and effective ways of treatment for yourself. As a patient, you can take control of your own health matters, with the guidance from your health care providers. You should feel free to ask any questions and expect to get unbiased answers. The decision to follow certain line of treatment should be ultimately taken by well-informed patient himself, who is willing to do efforts to overcome the disease. All this may not guarantee so called "cure "of any condition, but if combined with mainstream medicine, the results would be better than the present day health scenario.

CHAPTER 7

TREATMENT OF CANCER:
THE FOUNDATION

Last chapter explained the core, personality of the individual, which can greatly influence the outcome of any treatment. Negative emotions and thoughts hinder the recovery. Positive emotions, thoughts and will to get better help the recovery. It is usually difficult to radically change patterns of emotions and thoughts to support a healthier way of living. However, awareness of the importance of the power of own mind to overcome disease might provide a new direction for many people. This applies not only to cancer patients, but also to any ill person and even to all those who wish to prevent possible ill health. For healthy persons, tuning up the mind with positive thoughts might make life happier. A patient needs self-motivation as well as support from the family, friends and professionals in this matter. Mind-body medical techniques described earlier would help greatly for attending to the inner core.

Foundation of cancer treatment deals with:
1. Nutrition
2. Detoxification
3. Exercise, Deep Breathing, Massage, Yoga, Sleep
4. Social Support & Group Support

All these approaches are interlinked and sometimes overlap. Hence there is going to be repetition of some suggestions. It is best to attend to the foundation simultaneously with the main treatment for cancer. These methods are not directed against cancer cells, but aim at enabling your body to fight own battle. These are the support tools in the war. Without such support, the body would be unable to successfully continue the fight. These are like supply strategies to the war front.

NUTRITION:

Nutrition is much more than eating high protein diet with lots of vitamins. It is not enough to make a lot of goodies available. One has to be sure that all this nutrition can be properly consumed. It can be compared with a lot of pocket money given by a father to his school going child. Unless the child knows how to use the money properly, the generosity might prove worthless and even dangerous. A child with lot of money and little wisdom about how to spend it is more likely to end up in trouble. Same thing can happen with body. If the body is not able to digest, assimilate and convert all those nutrients, the effects of rich diet can be to produce more internal toxins and metabolic waste products. It is very important therefore to assess digestive capacity and assimilation powers of a person.

Digestion:
If digestion is weak, there is no use forcing good foods. Ayurved deals with concept of *Agni* in great details. Literally, agni means fire. In ayurvedic context, agni is the measure of digestive power of various organs, tissues and individual cells. Ayurved describes 13 sub-types of Agni. The main one is jathar-agni; jathar in Sanskrit stands for stomach. Agni in stomach is responsible for the appetite and for the digestion of the food. Good appetite at right time is the measure of jathar-agni. A person with normal agni would feel good hunger at mealtimes and will be satisfied after a normal meal. Lack of appetite indicates poor agni. Irregular appetite, variable from time to time, indicates imbalance in agni. False appetite, eating too much at a time and then developing acidity, flatulence and indigestion soon after meals are an indication of false agni. Besides the main jatharagni, other 12 agnis relate to functions of tissues and elements in the body. Poor appetite, flatulence, acidity, daytime napping, lack of enthusiasm are some of the pointers to the disturbed agni function. You need to see an Ayurvedic physician for medical management of this problem. However, following few simple instructions could be tried initially at home.

1. Do not overeat. Do not force food unless appetite improves. Too much food smothers agni, as too much wet wood smothers a fire.
2. If you can tolerate, skipping a meal might help to tune up agni. Weekly fasting may be another way of combining health benefits and rituals for the religiously oriented.
3. Take fruit juices, soups and light meals; rice, moong dal soup, boiled vegetables etc till appetite improves. You have to supplement such light diet with adequate vitamins and minerals. Avoid ice cold drinks, cold foods and stale foods.
4. Take a teaspoonful of a mixture of equal amounts of shredded fresh ginger, honey and lemon juice every morning. This could be repeated before each meal to stimulate agni.
5. Take a mild herbal laxative once in a while.
6. Vegetarian diet is preferable.

Assimilation & Elimination:
Once Agni is improved, assimilation of what you eat improves automatically. After absorption, the nourishment would be passed on to other tissue systems to be processed by their individual Agni. Slowly, you may start adding rich high protein diet. If assimilation were proper, the possibility of metabolic toxins accumulating in your system would be reduced. You would start feeling light, bright and cheerful.

A factory needs proper disposal of the waste products, which are generated during the process of manufacture. The body needs efficient elimination of waste products, which can become toxic if accumulated in body. Intestines, kidneys, skin, lungs and liver are the main organs for disposal. Keep them functioning properly. Unless advised by your doctor otherwise, drink lot of plain water, about 2 liters or more daily. This keeps body flushed and blood thin, which helps circulation. Kidneys can dispose some waste products better if more water is available. Moreover, cells can function better when adequate water is available. Remember, water constitutes more than 65% of body weight. Use of mild herbal laxatives and eating good quantity vegetables helps your bowel function well.

Nutrients to Protect Against Cancer:
Recent research has confirmed that nutrition plays a critical role in the causation as well as prevention of many diseases. Micronutrients are substances like vitamins, minerals, and enzymes etc, which are required in minute quantity for proper functioning of the cells. Modern food habits encourage over-consumption of empty calories that are high in fats and refined sugars but low in micronutrients. Such food habits impair natural immunity to diseases and lead to premature ageing. A diet should not be considered only as calories from fats, proteins and carbohydrates. Empty calories, devoid of any essential nutrients, could lead to many diseases apart from the apparent obesity! Modern agricultural techniques of liberal use of synthetic fertilizers, pesticides and other chemicals to increase the yield might reduce the quality of foods. Moreover, chemicals used in canning and other preservative techniques might introduce toxic products into our foods. Unable to deal with such foreign matter, body may store such toxins in various internal tissues. This would invite chronic ill health. Plant foods are richer sources of micronutrients. Ideally, all the calories and essential micronutrients should be obtained from fresh food, vegetables and fruits. In olden days, there was no awareness of vitamins, minerals and other supplements. People used to obtain all these nutrients, without knowing about the individual components, from traditional natural foods peculiar for their domiciles.

Vitamins and minerals help conversion of food to energy. Vitamin B complex and magnesium are "energy micronutrients" that activate enzymes. Enzymes are conductors of all biochemical reactions within cells. Vitamins A, C, E and minerals like zinc, copper, selenium, manganese are protector micronutrients that act together as a team to assist energy nutrients and to clear the cells of free radicals. Free radicals are liberated during all the metabolic activities of cells. Although needed for normal tissue functions, excessive free radicals can damage other molecules of cells and disturb their functions. This can lead to degenerative changes like heart disease, memory impairment, arthritis, cancer, premature ageing etc.

The quantity of unhealthy fats should be reduced from diet. However, it should be noted that good fats are essential for formation of cell walls and to help proper cell function. Essential fatty acids, like omega-3 and omega-6, AA, EPA, ALA, DHA should be taken in adequate amount to maintain good health. Flaxseed oil (linseed oil) is a good source of omega-3 fatty acids. Use of butter and pure ghee (clarified butter) in moderate quantities is recommended by Ayurveda for rejuvenation of cells, luster and energy. Similarly, proteins and essential amino acids are important for good health. Following is a list of some cancer preventive micronutrients:

1.Vitamin A: strengthens immune system. Essential for mineral metabolism and hormonal function. Helps detoxification of cells. This fat-soluble vitamin is found in fish oils, cod liver oil, butter and eggs.
2. Vitamin C: Important antioxidant that prevents damage from free radicals. Helps absorption of Vit A, iron and other micronutrients. Found in citrus fruits like oranges, apples, and lemons.
3. Vitamin B-6: Pyridoxine maintains health of mucous membranes. Fights infection and pollution. Protects against cancer. Found in bananas, green vegetables, carrots, apples and meats.
4. Vitamin D: required for strong bones. Protects against breast and colon cancer. Found in animal foods, butter, fish etc.
5. Vitamin E: Powerful antioxidant. Prevents tissue degeneration and ageing. Found in natural oils, wheat germs, and dark green vegetables. Essential to fight cancer.
6.Folic Acid: Needed for synthesis of healthy cells. Protects against cancer and heart attacks. Found in beets, cabbage, leafy vegetables, eggs, and dairy products.
7. Minerals: All minerals are needed for biochemical activities. Zinc, Selenium, magnesium and manganese are components of enzymes that help body fight cancer-producing toxins (carcinogens) and repair the damaged genes.
8. Lactic acid and Friendly Bacteria (probiotics): Normal friendly inhabitants of intestine. Help digest food and manufacture some

vitamins and micronutrients. Found in buttermilk, yogurts, curds, cheese and some lacto- fermented foods.

9. Co-Enzyme Q-10: Highly protective against cancer and heart diseases. Found in animal fats and nuts like pistachio.

10. Fiber: Whole grain fiber-rich foods are essential in any anti-cancer diet. Helps detoxification of intestinal toxins and elimination of waste products. Prevents colon cancer. Plentiful in grain husks and vegetables.

Foods To Avoid:
It is advisable to avoid foods made from white refined flour, white sugar, bakery products made from white flour, vanaspati ghee (hydrogenated vegetable oils), pop drinks, canned foods, foods containing artificial colors and chemical preservatives. Such processing techniques remove essential natural health promoting factors from the food. Cancer cells grow faster in acidic condition of cells. The above foods produce lot of acidity and indigestion. On the other hand, consumption of vegetables and fruits reduces the acidity in the body. That is why large amounts of vegetables and seasonal fruits in diet are very important for prevention and treatment of cancer.

General Advice:
It is difficult and probably unnecessary to focus the attention on individual micronutrients. A well-balanced natural diet containing seasonally available fresh vegetables, fruits and dairy products usually prevent many health problems including cancer. In certain specific situations, however, one may need to take high doses of individual cancer fighting micronutrients. Some doctors might advise against taking any vitamins and minerals during the course of chemotherapy and radiotherapy treatments. They might fear that such nutrients would promote growth of cancer cells, which they are trying to destroy. There are also fears that antioxidant supplements would counteract the free radicals liberated by radiotherapy and chemotherapy treatments, thereby reducing the effects of these anti-cancer treatments. Such fears are unfounded. Research done by Kedar Prasad at the University of Colorado and other scientists in USA, Japan and France has amply

demonstrated that supplements of micronutrients and antioxidants do not promote growth of cancer cells during radiotherapy and chemotherapy treatments. On the contrary, there are many reports indicating enhancement of action of chemotherapy drugs when additional vitamins and micronutrients are given simultaneously. Anyway, a doctor could not advise a patient not to eat fresh fruits, vegetables and healthy diet, which naturally contains all such micronutrients, antioxidants and vitamins. Hence, there should be no objection to supplement patient's diet with such micronutrients.

DETOXIFICATION:

Detoxification means removing toxic waste products from various parts of body. Nature has provided body with mechanisms of natural detoxifications. These are elimination of stools from intestine, urine from kidneys, sweat from skin, carbon dioxide from lungs etc. Liver is very important organ to remove biological and chemical toxins from blood. These are day-to-day elimination processes rather than what is implied by " detoxification" in alternative medicine.

Chronic exposure to pollutants and unhealthy foods liberate excessive amounts of certain chemicals unfamiliar to routine elimination channels. Heavy metals, industrial chemicals, pollutants in air, water and food are such examples. When faced with overload of toxins or due to unfamiliar nature of toxins, the body may be unable to cope up with such toxins. The toxins keep accumulating in the body. The body stores such unwanted guests in secondary sites such as muscles, fats, bones etc. Some toxic substances have tendency to accumulate in critical organs like liver, heart, brain and kidneys. Obviously, such toxic storehouses would lead to chronic and acute health problems. In acute illness, body works hard to dispose such toxins. When the body succeeds, acute episode of illness is over. If body is unable to deal with such a problems, a disease turns chronic. It is a low level warfare, a sort of cold war. It is there but may not put you out of work. You get "used to it", if you will! This is the beginning of chronic diseases. Cancer starts in this fashion chronically. Hence, there are hopes to reverse the process and win the battle against cancer.

Caution:
General information is given below about certain detoxification methods. This is for the information only and you should not undertake any of these methods on your own without consulting a knowledgeable health care provider. This has to be done under medical supervision. If wrongly performed, these methods could be harmful to your health.

Detoxification Methods:
Most of the alternative medical systems and even allopathic medicine believe in detoxifications. Allopathic medicine has special protocols to deal with various poisons. In overdose toxicity of some drugs, intravenous infusions of n-acetyl cystein are recommended to enable liver to remove such toxins. For heavy metal poisoning, chelation therapy, which consists of infusions of EDTA (ethylene-diamine- tetra acetic acid), has been advocated. In overdoses of pharmaceutical drugs and drug reactions, intravenous infusions to promote elimination of toxins through kidney are routinely used.

Ayurvedic *Pancha-karma*:
Various methods of alternative medicine advocate their own brands of detoxification methods. This is called purification of body in Ayurveda. Pancha-karma, a vital modality in Ayurveda, deals in details with five fold purification techniques. Pancha-karma literally means five procedures. Ayurveda states that a disturbed *dosha* gets accumulated in body and leads to disease. A body has three dosha, which are basic constituents that are liable to get disturbed. To eradicate a specific dosha, a specific type of *karma* (procedure) is advised. Vata, Pitta and Kapha are three doshas, which are responsible to cause disease. Vaman, Virechan, Basti, Nasya and Shirodhara are five basic pancha-karma described in Ayurvedic texts for dealing with accumulated dosha. These have to be undertaken by an experienced Ayurvedic practitioner.

Pancha –karma are especially recommended as a basic cleaning procedure in dealing with chronic diseases. I have personally witnessed improvement in general condition and relief of painful symptoms even in advanced cancer patients. It is not a curative treatment for cancer but it certainly helps to balance body functions. Pancha-karma is an intensive detoxification/ purification strategy to be done only under supervision of an experienced Ayurvedic physician. In addition to pancha-karma, Ayurveda prescribes various oral herbal medicines to stimulate functions of liver, kidney, skin, lungs and bowel.

Fasting:
Proper digestion, assimilation and elimination are nature's methods of detoxification. All the good nutritional practices described earlier would help detoxification. Fasting is known to stimulate Agni and burn up accumulated *Aama*, an internal metabolic toxin described by Ayurveda. Various versions of abstaining from solid foods and consumption of vegetable and fruit juices have been developed in different parts of the world as a part of treatment of chronic diseases.

Intestinal Toxicity:
Many chronic illnesses such as cancer, allergies, infections, liver diseases, skin diseases etc might start in the intestines. When the intestines become clogged by poor habits of digestion and elimination, toxicity develops. The waste products stagnate and putrefy. These toxins are absorbed through the intestines and reach other parts of the body. This can create acute as well as chronic health problems. Current age of fast foods is having a bad impact on people, especially on the younger generation. Old healthy habits are looked down upon as backward behavior. In a busy city, parents and children have little time or inclination to eat a healthy meal at home. In young age, the body somehow copes up. Over the long run, these habits lead to chronic health problems. Foods made of white flour, white sugar are difficult to digest. Lack of adequate vegetables in diet may lead to chronic constipation. That is why timely elimination of bowel is of utmost importance for good health. It is the duty of parents to enforce good food habits upon the children, not by talk alone but by self-example.

Colonics and Enemas:

Some alternative medical centers around the world use repeated colonic irrigations to cleanse the bowel. They believe that this is a good way to remove the toxins from body. I do not know if such an intensive cleansing is beneficial or tolerable for an average person. Coffee enema uses decoction of ground coffee beans as a fluid introduced and retained in colon. Coffee, it is claimed, gets absorbed and goes to the liver to improve the liver function and help the liver to remove the toxins in blood. I personally would not recommend any intensive frequent colonics. I believe mild herbal laxatives, as per the needs, would suffice for an average person. You should follow the advice of your doctors in this matter. There is a danger of dehydration (loss of vital water from the body) in such intensive colonics. Occasional patient might benefit by enema, but this should be done under medical supervision.

Homeopathy For Detoxification:

Homeopathy uses natural substances in different dilutions to treat health problems. Dilutions are termed as homeopathic potencies. A peculiar way of preparation of homeopathic products imparts potencies to the remedies. Higher the dilution, higher is the potency. We will try to explain homeopathy in greater details in a later chapter. Recently, combinations of certain homeopathic remedies in low potencies are being given to patients to improve the functions of organs responsible for detoxification. These target organs are mainly liver, kidney, skin, lung, bowel and lung. Homeopathic combinations in low potencies are called drainage remedies, which improve the draining capacity of target organs. After tuning up such target organs with drainage remedies, the next step is to use other specific remedies for homeopathic detoxification. This approach helps to move accumulated toxins from different parts of the body for disposal through specific organs. These toxins could be metabolic internal toxins or could be external chemicals and heavy metals, which have accumulated in the body over a period of time. When the drainage organs are tuned up for optimal function, these loose circulating toxins are easily removed from the body. If drainage is not optimal then these loose toxins, instead of getting out of the system, re-circulate and can cause various side reactions. Hence, homeopathic detoxification has to be undertaken under proper medical supervision.

Massage Therapy & Skin Detoxification:

Proper cleanliness and regular bathing is important for skin detoxification. Air pollution, dust and use of chemical deodorants, cosmetics etc can clog the skin pores. This is dangerous for skin health. Skin is the largest surface of the body, which can eliminate a lot of toxins through sweating. Artificial attempts to stop perspiration should be discouraged. According to Ayurveda, skin is an organ responsible for balance of *Vata Dosha*. You might need to take whole body oil massage weekly followed by hot water bath to keep the skin pores open and functioning well. Simple Coconut oil, til (sesame) oil or olive oil can be used for body massage. The massage stimulates various energy points (termed as acupressure points in Chinese medicine or marma-points in Ayurveda). This establishes proper flow of prana-energy throughout body. Ayurveda and yoga describe nadis; energy channels, throughout the body. Massage stimulates blood circulation. Massage has been proved beneficial in various chronic health problems.

Deep Breathing and Lung Detoxification:

Two time Nobel laureate, Dr Otto Warburg from Germany proved that lack of oxygen can change normal cells to become cancerous. He proved that normal embryo cells grown in laboratory petri dish turn cancerous when deprived of oxygen. Oxygen is important for all the activities of body. Oxygen acting within each cell provides energy for the life.

The technique of breathing is critical for physical and psychological health. Most of us breath shallow and superficial. This is chest breathing where with each incoming breath, only ribs move outward allowing very limited quantity of fresh air to enter in the lungs. Most of us are not aware of our breathing and we breathe too rapidly, especially under stress. Deep abdominal breathing can double or triple our supply of oxygen to our blood. This technique is simple to learn but must be practiced sincerely for long time to get health benefits. Diaphragm is the strong muscle separating lungs above from abdomen below. In shallow breathing, diaphragm does not move much. If diaphragm is moved consciously up and down during deep breathing, this act can ventilate lungs with fresh air about two to three times more. A shallow breath will exchange about 500 cc (one half liter) of air. A deep abdominal breath can exchange about 1500 to 2000 cc of fresh air in each cycle. A deep breath can ventilate your deepest folds of lungs. When the lungs expand fully, more oxygen can go in to purify the blood and at the same time impure gases like carbon dioxide etc can be removed easily.

Lymph is the tissue fluid surrounding all the cells of our body. Lymph is not blood. Lymph circulates through smaller lymph vessels, which run parallel to blood vessels. The biggest store of lymph, *cysterna chili*, is below diaphragm near liver and stomach. Strong movements of diaphragm help to pump up the lymph towards aorta where it eventually mixes with blood circulation. Lymph circulation is very important for cellular health. Lymph takes care of all the supply needs of individual cells. Lymph also helps to remove toxins and germs.

Deep breathing helps to stabilize our mind. The mind becomes more focused and concentrated. A concentrated mind is peaceful and powerful. It is our everyday experience that deep breathing can tranquilize our agitated mind. Deep breathing thus helps for our emotional detoxification. Harmful emotions like anger, anxiety, lust, greed etc could be controlled with a peaceful tranquil mind.

To learn deep abdominal breathing, lie down flat on your back on ground or on a firm bed. Watch your breathing. Evaluate if your breathing is regular. Put palm of one hand on your belly and feel if the belly moves up and down with the breathing. When you breathe in, the belly should come up and when you breathe out, the belly should recede back. The movement of the belly during breathing is the indicator of deep breathing. If the belly is not moving much, try to move it out when you take a deep breath in and try to bring it in when you breathe out. Diaphragm is pulled down when you take in a deep breath and belly comes forward. When you breathe out, the diaphragm moves up and belly comes in. Repeat this few times daily. Once you learn this technique, it can be practiced in any position and at any time of the day. By repeated practice, one should be able to learn deep abdominal breathing within few days. Whenever you get time, consciously practice deep breathing. Eventually, this should become a habit. You will be breathing more slowly but more deeply. You could also learn this technique from a yoga practitioner.

Exercise:
Exercise is very important for energy, circulation, detoxification and good health. Some of us will love to do vigorous exercise like weight lifting and other gymnastics. Some of us will be happy with running, jogging or even walking. You have to find your own suitable exercise, which is comfortable and invigorating for you. Regularity is most important. For most of us, brisk walking for 30 to 40 minutes daily is sufficient. This kind of exercise, which can be easily performed anywhere, will raise your heartbeats, stretch your muscles, ventilate your lungs, circulate your blood and help remove accumulated toxins. The muscles become strong. Regular exercise has been shown to improve your immunity, a fact that is confirmed by appropriate laboratory tests. You might need to talk to a physiotherapist or other health care professional if you have any questions about your exercise schedules.

Yoga:
In Sanskrit, Yoga means "Union", Yuj= to unite. Yoga has a very special place in India. Practice of yoga has physical, psychological as well as spiritual benefits. Yoga describes higher techniques of *pranayama*, controlling the breath, which can be learnt after getting used to deep abdominal breathing. The type of yoga seen on TV or taught in classes is mostly physical activities and specific postures. This physical yoga too definitely has lot of health benefits. More subtle types of yoga consist of steady postures, *pranayama, dhyan, dharana* and ultimately *samadhi*. Yoga has to be practiced under the guidance of trained teachers or Guru. Practice of yoga can improve physiological as

well as psychological functions. Various *aasana* and *mudra* used in yoga can direct the flow of vital energy. Specific postures of *aasana and mudra* can direct the energy to deficient internal organs that require the boost. Besides physical benefits, practice of yoga can provide peace, tranquility and mental energy to overcome problems in life.

Movement Therapy:
Synchronous body movements are known to balance internal energy, improve circulation of lymph and blood, help mental concentration and produce relaxation. Dance is a type of movement therapy. Dance therapy is a good example of combining movement therapy, recreation and exercise. Group dances as practiced in western culture offer many benefits. Such dances can be considered as combinations of group therapy, exercise therapy, psychotherapy, hypnotherapy etc. There are various dance rituals in primitive tribal societies. Many such rituals are practiced by the medicine men of old cultures. Many different schools of Indian classical dances have evolved over many centuries. Indian classical dance, unlike western group dance, requires years of rigorous practice and devotion to become an accomplished dancer. Undoubtedly, such highly evolved classical dances bestow health benefits apart from the main objective of creative art to enrich the life.

Qigong:
Qigong (pronounced as chee gung) is an ancient movement therapy evolved in China. With gentle, rhythmic movements, a person could direct the vital energy (Qi) through various meridians, energy channels in the body. In China, there are over 100 million people estimated to practice Qigong regularly. Qigong is offered in various hospitals and medical clinics across China as a complementary therapy for various diseases. Qigong has to be learnt from trained teachers and practitioners of this art.

Sleep:
In a true sense, sleep is not a therapy but is the basic necessity of life. Without proper sleep, normal activities of the life are impossible. As the day cannot be imagined without the night, waking life cannot be

imagined without sleep. People are ready to do anything to get a good night's sleep. Sleep heals the harmful changes produced by activities of life. It helps healing of cells, restore peace of mind, and freshen up the organs to continue daily battle for survival. Deep sleep has been shown to restore immune functions. There is a small gland called pineal gland, about the size of a peanut, in the center of the brain. This mysterious gland is a part of endocrine system. Endocrine glands secrete hormones required for important functions in body. Other members of endocrine system that secrete hormones are pituitary, thyroid, adrenal, ovaries, testes, and pancreas. Hormones are very powerful minute secretions, which circulate in blood and control critical functions of other organs of the body. The significance of pineal hormones is not yet fully understood. Melatonin is one hormone known to be secreted by the pineal gland. Brain melatonin levels rise dramatically at night. It is a sleep-promoting hormone. Melatonin also appears to have a substantial cancer repelling activity. It boosts activity of key immune cells viz lymphocytes, T-cells, natural killer cells and stimulate production cytokine interleukins-2. All these are immune components required to fight cancer and many other diseases. Gentle massage to head and soles of feet, soothing music, quiet surroundings, light diet can all help to invite sound sleep. Of course there are sleeping pills, but these pharmacological drugs usually produce artificial sleep with some unpleasant side effects on waking. Certain homeopathic remedies, such as Kali-phos and Ignatia can sometimes pacify the mental agitations and thus help to get gentle sleep. Any such remedies should be taken with proper consultation with a health practitioner.

Hobbies:
You should try to devote some time to any hobby that suits you. Games, music, singing, reading, writing, drama, dance, travel, chit-chatting, chanting, painting and even cooking are the examples of some recreative hobbies. Such hobbies tend to occupy the mind constructively and life becomes cheerful and worth living. Hobbies provide relaxation, cheerfulness and could be of great help in fighting diseases.

Relaxation:

Relaxation is very important for stress reduction. Various hobbies help one relax. Good thoughts and cultivation of positive mental attitudes is very helpful for good health.

Relaxation Response, a term coined by Dr Herbert Benson of Boston, is a meditation technique without any religious overtones. Dr. Benson has proved that concentrating on any sound, repeatedly in a certain fashion, can produce relaxation of body and mind. This can offer highly significant health benefits.

Social Support:

Man is a social animal. We all need support from family and friends. Feelings of isolation, rejection, hopelessness, despair etc are detrimental for health and happiness. Psychotherapy and group therapy help one to ventilate personal fears, doubts, and insecurities. This goes a long way to improve mental health, which in turn will help one to get over the physical health problems. One should seek company of kind sympathetic and helpful friends and relatives. One should have some sympathetic ear available. Even if some problems cannot be solved, mere bringing them out in open is itself a treatment. Many times, a positive mind successfully finds healthy ways to react to these trying circumstances.

Group Therapies:

Exceptional cancer patients who have overcome their cancer have started many groups for cancer patients. Sharing personal experiences and concerns benefits all the members of such groups. One should feel free to discuss any concerns and questions with own doctors. One can take help from psychologist and social workers to find out about psychotherapy and group therapy. Breast cancer support groups are very common, which have been started by motivated breast cancer patients. David Spiegel, a psychiatrist at Stanford University, demonstrated that women with breast cancer who participated in a weekly support group lived twice as long as those who did not. In majority of studies reporting significant improvement in survival of cancer patients, patients were involved in psychotherapy and supportive group therapy.

Conclusion:

This chapter described certain tools, which you can learn and practice. Practicing these would certainly impart health benefits. You would be in a better position to improve your health and happiness. The core and the foundation of the treatment described in this and earlier chapter should be put in practice as soon as possible, possibly even before or simultaneously with other definitive treatment for cancer you might choose to undergo. Please feel free to discuss all your concerns and questions with your health care providers. Please remember that you could and should help in a great way in your own health care. Take an informed decision. Be an equal partner in your own health care.

Chapter 8

Conventional Treatment:
Surgery, Radiotherapy, Chemotherapy

As soon as diagnosis of cancer is announced, there is immediate rush for starting the treatment. Naturally, everyone wishes to extricate this enemy from the body as soon as possible. Surgery, Radiotherapy and Chemotherapy are the mainstay of the conventional treatment. The doctor should discuss various treatment options and possible outcome with the patient and the relatives. This would give a chance to the patient to understand possible benefits and risks of suggested treatment methods. It is commonly seen that doctors recommend a particular line of treatment but might not give adequate explanation about possible limitations and side effects of such treatment. Patients usually believe that once the recommended treatment is taken, the cure would follow. It is important for the patient and for the relatives to obtain all the information about the efficacy, safety, risks and costs about any recommended treatment.

A considerate doctor, either a family physician or a specialist, can help greatly to discuss these issues and prepare the patient for a proper line of treatment. Such discussions, before undertaking a course of treatment, would go a long way to help the patient complete the treatment course without undue anxiety. Only a small number of patients feel free to ask all the information they need to know in this matter. Most of the doctors are willing to answer all the questions of the patients. In India, majority of the patients feel shy or scared to ask too many questions fearing displeasure of the doctors. Patients are eager to start treatment as soon as possible and might feel that critical time would be wasted in asking questions. I would suggest that each person should freely ask all the questions, however trivial these might appear. Time spent in getting all the information is time well spent. This might minimize doubts, anxieties and insecurities, which are likely to arise during the long course of cancer treatment. A patient should also simultaneously attend to the core and fundamentals of cancer treatment described earlier, which is essential to get better results and to reduce the risk of failure.

Before deciding the treatment, your doctors will need to carry out certain blood tests, X-rays, Scans etc to outline exact location, size and spread of cancer. Individual treatment would depend upon the findings from such tests. In order to withstand any major treatments, your general condition and strength should be adequate. Old age is no bar for surgery.

Surgery:

Surgery is still the gold standard of cancer treatment. Contrary to the common public perception, surgery is not the last resort. Surgery is effective in localized cancer tumors, which have not spread to lymph nodes or distant organs. Complete surgical removal of the tumor, when possible, improves the chances of cure. Results of surgery are different in different types of cancer. Not every type of cancer can be controlled by the surgery. Following is only a brief description of some basic surgical procedures. This is a very wide subject and there are many individual variations. It is best to discuss all the details with the surgeon likely to perform the operation on the patient.

Radical Surgery, usually a major operation, removes the entire tumor together with nearby lymph nodes that are likely to harbor displaced cancer cells. Modern techniques of anesthesia, operative skills, life support during surgery and efficient recovery rooms make even long complicated major operations safe.

Radical surgery for cancer in head, neck, mouth or throat is routinely performed. Such major operations usually lead to disfigurement of face. Many patients accept such operation hoping for cure. Many times, such operations can cause a lot of emotional stress besides physical difficulties in critical functions such as speaking and swallowing. One should discuss about all these possible merits and demerits and then take informed decision.

Palliative Surgery is performed when complete removal of tumor is not possible. Palliative surgery is considered if such an operation can provide relief to the suffering of the patient. Palliative surgery is done to reduce pain, pressure or interference with critical function hoping to improve the quality of remaining life. Such operations are less extensive than radical operations, less strenuous for the patient but not aimed to cure the cancer. Sometimes a large tumor, or part of it, is removed to relieve pressure and obstruction of the tumor on critical organs. At other times, a large tumor is removed leaving smaller parts of cancer behind that can be dealt with radiotherapy and / or chemotherapy.

Diversion Procedures:
When a patient is unable to breathe due to tumor obstruction in throat or due to radiation reaction, tracheostomy is performed. This is placing a tube in the trachea, the windpipe in neck. This procedure is simple to do but could prove very uncomfortable for the patient, later on. This should be done only when severe breathing difficulty actually develops and not routinely. Many times, breathing difficulties can be dealt with simpler non-surgical treatments.

Gastrostomy/ Jejunostomy: When a patient is unable to swallow food due to cancer pressing the food-pipe, a rubber or plastic tube is introduced within the stomach or intestines through the front of the abdomen. Liquid foods can thus be introduced through the tube bypassing the mouth and food-pipe. This simple procedure helps to supply the needed nourishment to the patient for some period. Gastrostomy does not remove the tumor; it only provides a diversion.

Colostomy is another common procedure performed to divert stools. When stools cannot pass normally due to tumor obstructing in rectum, external opening is made in lower part of abdomen to divert the passage of stools. This simple but troublesome procedure is usually done under local anesthesia.

When urine flow is obstructed due to tumor in urethra or due to non-functioning of urinary bladder, a rubber or plastic catheter is passed through urethra upwards to provide an outlet for stagnated urine. This is called a urinary catheterization.

Doctors should discuss with the patients all the possible benefits as well as possible problems associated with various lines of treatments. Patients have to consider all such possible benefits and possible problems and then give their consent for such treatments.

Radiotherapy:

Radiotherapy means treatment with radiation energy. X-ray is a type of man-made radiation energy. X-rays were discovered around 1895. During initial enthusiasm, X-rays were used to treat many diseases. As the time went by, limitations and risks of radiation treatments were being understood more clearly. Around same time, Madam Curie discovered radioactivity. Radium was put to medical use for various conditions. As the science advanced, many more radioactive materials were discovered, some natural and many man made in nuclear reactors. X rays and radioactive alpha, beta and gamma rays are examples of ionizing radiation.

These invisible radiations cause bio-chemical changes in cells. In low doses, radiation leads to mutations, changes in genes- the code of life. Radiation energy, in high doses, can destroy cells. On the earth, we are all constantly exposed to very minute doses of natural radiations from the Sun, from the atmosphere and even from the earth. For medical uses of radiation energy, strict controls and safety procedures are enforced by various government agencies. X-rays and radioactive materials are used to treat certain medical conditions. This branch is called Therapeutic Radiology or Radiotherapy. Currently, radiotherapy is mostly restricted to the treatment of malignant conditions.

Radiation Machines:
Earlier, Superficial and Deep X-ray therapy machines were commonly used to give radiation. X-rays are generated when high voltage electrical current is passed through a vacuum tube, called as X-Ray Tube. Voltages less than 100 kilovolts produce superficial x-rays while 100 to 300 kilovolts produce deep x-rays of variable strength. Higher the voltage used, deeper the penetration of x-rays in the body.

Cobalt machines have a small 2 cm diameter powerful source of radioactive cobalt, which constantly emits high-energy gamma rays. Through special arrangements, a radiation beam of required size can be directed at the cancer area in the patient.

Linear Accelerators are latest expensive radiation machines that generate very powerful x-rays at voltages ranging from 4 to 20 million volts (mega volts). These radiations penetrate deeply to reach deep-seated tumors, which are beyond the reach of deep x-rays or cobalt rays. Linear accelerators can also emit high voltage electrons, which are energy particles rather than waves like gamma rays or x-rays. High voltage electrons have a special use in treatment of superficial cancer.

How Radiation Works:
Cancer cells have larger nuclei and they divide more rapidly than normal cells. This makes them more vulnerable to be destroyed by radiation. However, normal tissues and organs coming in the way of radiation beam would develop some damage. This results in radiation reactions. Over a period of few weeks, acute radiation reactions subside, but some chronic changes are left behind permanently.

X-rays, gamma rays and electrons pass through body. Tissues and cells coming in the way of radiation beam absorb part of the radiation energy. This absorbed energy causes chemical changes in cells and damage to chromosomes. A sufficient dose of radiation energy would deeply affect the cells, which become unable to function or to divide. When cells are unable to multiply that is called cell death. When most of the cancer cells die, tumor shrinks and cancer is said to be under control (remission).

The doctors closely monitor a patient under radiotherapy. Necessary changes are made to radiation plans as per individual needs. Supportive medicines are prescribed to reduce the radiation reactions. If the reactions are severe, radiotherapy is suspended for few days for recovery of normal cells.

Brachytherapy:

Application of radiotherapy beam from outside to a part of body is called teletherapy. Tele means from a distance. Use of X-rays, Cobalt Rays and Linear Accelerators are examples of teletherapy. Brachytherapy is a radiotherapy technique wherein radiation is given from within the body. Small radioactive needles or seeds are implanted or inserted within the cancer tumor by a surgical procedure. Some implants are removable after certain number of hours; others are permanent implants wherein the small seeds of radioactive isotope are left permanently within cancer area. The dose and intensity of radiation varies greatly with the type of implant. Brachytherapy is very important for cancers of uterus, mouth and breast. Brachytherapy delivers high doses to a very limited tumor area around the implant. Careful planning needs to be done to avoid excessive doses of radiation that can lead to long-term damage to surrounding normal organs.

Radio-neuro-surgery:

Brain tumors need to be removed by neuro-surgical operations. In the last few years, a new technique called gamma-knife or X-knife has become available. For small tumors located deep within brain, computer assisted external radiation beams are able to deliver very high doses of radiation to the exact shape and size of tumor seen on scans. Results are similar to surgical removal of small tumors. This treatment causes total destruction of the tumor area hence termed as radio-neuro-surgery. Precise planning and proper case selection is necessary for application of these expensive techniques.

Scope of Radiotherapy:
Radiotherapy is used in more than 60 % to 70 % cancer patients. Radiotherapy can be used for short-term palliation of symptoms or it could be used as a curative radical treatment. In radical treatment, higher doses of radiation are given hoping to cure the cancer while accepting more side reactions. Radiotherapy can also be planned as a pre-operative or post-operative course to supplement the surgical treatment of cancer. Radiotherapy can also be used in adjuvant fashion together with chemotherapy courses. There are various permutations and combinations of Surgery, Radiotherapy and Chemotherapy as per the specific needs of the situation. When combined, the effectiveness of the treatment increases but at the same time the possibility of damage to normal organs also increases.

Radiotherapy is useful to control cancers of mouth, throat, uterus, and some low-grade brain tumors and lymph node cancers. Cancers of stomach, intestines, colon, liver, pancreas, lung, kidney, sarcoma etc cannot be cured by radiation. When cancer is widely spread, radiotherapy may usually provide temporary local pain relief from painful metastases. Doctors weigh the possible benefits against possible risks of such combinations and advise the patient accordingly. Good general condition, belief in the treatment and positive optimistic attitude help the patient to derive more benefits out of such treatments.

Radiotherapy Course:
Detailed radiation planning is done before starting radiotherapy treatments to make sure that precise dose of radiation is administered to the tumor area. Each radiation treatment lasts for only a few minutes. During radiation treatment, patient does not feel any sensation of pain, shock or electric current. Radiation is administered in multiple small fractions. This reduces side effects and gives time for normal cells to recover.

After completion of radiotherapy course, doctors will review your case records and issue a report about your response. Thereafter you will be advised to see your doctors for regular check-ups. A good number of localized early stage cancers can be controlled with radiation alone. However, if cancer does not respond or if it comes back, you will be advised to see other specialists for surgery, chemotherapy etc.

Side Effects and Reactions:
Radiation reactions are acute or chronic, severe or mild, short term or long term. General reactions like loss of appetite, nausea, vomiting, lack of energy, and increased heat in body are common. Reactions start appearing within few days and go on increasing as the treatment progresses. The peak of reactions is usually around 3rd and 4th week of radiotherapy. Thereafter, the reactions usually start subsiding.

Local reactions depend upon the body area under radiotherapy. Patient who is receiving radiotherapy on mouth, throat and neck develops difficulty in swallowing due to inflammation. There could be burning sensation. Spicy foods irritate. Voice could be disturbed due to effect on voice box. Irritation of air passage can cause dry painful cough. Radiation on abdomen can cause severe vomiting and abdominal cramps. Patient could develop continued dull pains if inflammation affects internal organs. Radiation on chest might cause difficulty in breathing and difficulty in swallowing. There could be local pain and burning. Treatment on brain can cause headache, congestion and loss of hair. Treatment on lower abdomen and pelvis can cause urinary burning, painful diarrhea and piles. There are many other less common reactions.

While under radiotherapy, feel free to express your concerns and ask questions. The doctors will attend to your problems and do the needful to minimize your suffering. You should continue to have supplements of vitamins, minerals and some specific medications to help you during radiotherapy course. It is advisable to take extra doses of natural vitamin E, Vitamin C by mouth and injections of high dose vitamin B complex during course of radiotherapy and chemotherapy. If you were constipated, it would be advisable to take mild herbal laxatives periodically. You should consult your doctor for the details. In general, drink a lot of plain water, eat light easy to digest food, avoid constipation, have faith in the treatment and feel free to ask questions. Take the prescribed medications on time.

Chemotherapy:

Chemotherapy means treatment with chemicals. It is a general term but in the context of cancer, it implies use of drugs to destroy cancer cells. Such drugs are called cyto-toxic meaning poisonous to cells. Some drugs are cytostatic, which prevent cells from multiplying rather than causing direct cell death. Cancer cells grow faster and in chaotic fashion. Chemotherapy drugs are given either orally or by injection. Some drugs can be applied on body surface or injected directly into tumor area. In general, chemotherapy drugs destroy cancer cells more easily than normal cells. Normal cells are less damaged by chemotherapy drugs and recover faster than cancer cells.

Chemotherapy drugs act at various levels of cell growth. Some drugs disrupt mitosis, the actual process of new cell formation. Some drugs interfere with synthesis of nucleic acid that is required for formation of DNA and RNA molecules. Still other drugs act at multiple steps in the cell cycle. Mechanism of action of some drugs is still uncertain.

Chemotherapy Drugs:
Modern chemotherapy started with use of Nitrogen Mustard, a poisonous gas used in the Second World War. Soon, many other chemotherapy drugs were developed after extensive research and clinical trials. There are various classes of chemotherapy drugs. Following table lists some common chemotherapy drugs and their possible action. This list is not exhaustive and newer drugs are being continuously added. The list is given only for a general information and should not be used as a guide for self-treatment. Chemotherapy is a very complex subject and should be done only by the experienced doctors specially trained in this branch of medicine.

LIST OF SOME COMMONLY USED CHEMOTHERAPEUTIC DRUGS

CLASS	NAME	ACTION
Alkylating Agents	Nitrogen Mustard, Cytoxan, Endoxan Clorambucil, Thiotepa, Melphalan, Busulphan,	Damage DNA and Chromosomes
Platinum Compounds	Cisplatin, Carboplatin	Same as above
Antitumor antibiotics	Adriamycin, Epirubicin, Bleomycin, Actinomycin-D, Mitomycin-C	Same as above
Antimetabolites	Fluoro-uracil, Methotrexate, Hydroxyurea, L-asperginase	Interfere nucleic acid synthesis
Mitotic Spindle Inhibitors	Vinca alkaloids (Vincristin, Vinblastin), Paclitaxel	Inhibit tubulin and disrupts mitosis
Miscellaneous	Dacarbazine, Procarbazine etc.	Uncertain mechanism

Scope of Chemotherapy:
As stated by Dr. S. Eckhardt, M.D. of National Cancer Institute, (UICC Manual of Clinical Oncology, Fifth Edition, page 122), "Chemotherapy has proven to be curative in certain rare neoplastic diseases which represent approximately 5 % of all cancers. In commonly encountered types of cancers, however, chemotherapy has been less effective."

Although routinely prescribed in majority of cancer patient, chemotherapy is reported to cure only a small fraction of all cancers. UICC Manual of Clinical Oncology, Fifth Edition, page132, lists types of cancer, which can possibly be cured by chemotherapy. These are:

1. Choriocarcinoma, Leukemia in children
2. Acute Lymphocytic
3. Hodgekin's disease
4. Malignant Lymphoma
5. Testicular cancer, germ type
6. Ovarian cancer
7. Wilm's tumor, kidney cancer in children
8. Embryonal rhabdomyosarcoma
9. Ewing's sarcoma
10. Acute Myeloid Leukemia in adults

On page 131, the manual further states, " Of patients treated yearly with chemotherapy, possibly 20 % have curable disease and additional 20 % may experience significant prolongation of life. The remaining 60% have minimal or no benefit from cytostatic treatment and suffer from its toxic side reactions."

Chemotherapy Course:
When chemotherapy is prescribed after treatment with surgery and/ or radiotherapy, it is called as adjuvant chemotherapy. The object of adjuvant chemotherapy is minimizing chances of recurrence of cancer. Chemotherapy can be given as a single drug, but more often it is given as combination of two or more drugs to increase the effect and reduce the toxicity. This is called as combination chemotherapy and it is the most commonly used current pattern. Various combinations and protocols have evolved to deal with various situations. Palliative chemotherapy is used to relieve the patient of pain and some distressing problems related to cancer. Palliative chemotherapy is used for a short term and with reduced doses, not expecting a cure.

Chemotherapy course is usually given in a number of cycles extending over a period of weeks or months. Gap between each individual cycle is essential to enable body to recover from the side reactions of previous cycle. Before each cycle, careful assessment and blood tests are done by the medical oncoligists prescribing such chemotherapy cycles. If the reactions are too severe and if general condition is too weak, chemotherapy cycles are postponed. Special medicines and supplements are given to reduce avoidable side effects.

Chemotherapy Side Effects and Reactions:
Side effects and reactions are a dreaded subject for cancer patients. Although chemotherapy drugs are unable to distinguish normal cells from cancer cells, rapidly dividing cancer cells are usually killed in greater numbers than the normal cells. When the normal cells and organs suffer damage, reactions occur. Body's rapidly dividing cells found in bone marrow, mouth, stomach, intestines and hair follicles bear the brunt of the damage. Anemia and loss of white blood cells result from effect on bone marrow. Sores in mouth, throat and pile like symptoms are common. Ulcers in stomach and intestine might be painful and liable to bleed. Nausea, vomiting, loss of appetite, diarrhea, constipation, lack of energy, loss of sleep and suppressed immunity with risk of infections are common general side effects. Other side effects might include neurological problems, skin rashes, problems of lung, kidney and liver. Not all the chemotherapy drugs have same toxic side effects. Different drugs have different sites of reactions. Certain preventive medicines used simultaneously might reduce these side effects to variable degree. In young children, where the cells are rapidly growing, the side effects of chemotherapy may be more severe.

There are no fixed rules to avoid the side effects of chemotherapy. Proper nutritional support including Vitamins A, B Complex, C, D and E are important to help body to recover faster. Minerals like calcium, magnesium, zinc, selenium, manganese and trace elements are required for the cells to recover faster. A mixture of shredded ginger, lemon and honey in equal amounts taken a spoonful at a time reduces nausea associated with chemotherapy. Certain Ayurvedic preparations help to reduce the body heat experienced during chemotherapy. Many herbs, dietary supplements and homeopathic remedies are known to reduce side effects of chemotherapy. You need to consult the respective doctors for advice in this matter.

If you are advised to undergo chemotherapy, you should have a detailed discussion with the oncologist about possible benefits and possible hazards. Feel free to ask any questions. Do not feel threatened with the diagnosis of cancer. Big "C" need not force you to make a choice in hurry without getting all the information for the right decision. Take a decision wisely, especially if the benefits of chemotherapy are not certain. Cancer treatments, especially chemotherapy, could be an expensive affair. Although considered a bad word in modern medical treatment, "cost benefit ratio" has to be considered, especially when you have to spend your hard-earned money.

Hormone Therapy:

Hormones are very minute but powerful secretions from various internal glands within the body. Hormones control functions of organs and cells. Two thirds of cancers of prostate and a third of cancers of breast are dependent on hormone for growth. Estrogen, the female hormone, stimulates growth of breast cancers in some women. Similarly, androgen, the male hormone, stimulates the growth of prostate cancers in some men. Hormones and anti-hormones have been tried in treatment of such cancers.

Tamoxifen, a synthetic antiestrogen, is routinely given to patients of breast cancer. Flutamide, a drug working against androgen, is employed for prostate cancer. The response is variable and depends upon the presence of specific hormone receptors in the cancer cells. Certain tests are usually performed before prescribing such hormonal treatments. Progesterone, another hormone secreted by ovary, is sometimes useful for cancers of uterus and ovary. Corticosteroids, hormones from adrenal glands, are given for patients of leukemia and lymphoma. Hormonal treatment requires careful patient assessment by an experienced oncologist.

Immunotherapy:

Ideally, immunotherapy would be the best answer to cure cancer, since cancer is caused by decreased immunity. Immunotherapy, however, is a complex subject and defies easy solutions. There are many types of immune cells. Immunity is not one single unit. Different diseases might have different immunological deficiencies, most of which are yet poorly understood. An otherwise healthy individual may develop cancer due to lack of only a specific part of immunity.

Vaccines are prepared from weakened germs and their toxins. These are injected to give immunity in many diseases such as small pox, chicken pox, measles, mumps, cholera, typhoid, tetanus, diphtheria etc. Cancer is not due to a particular germ; hence a specific vaccine cannot be developed for cancer. However, many vaccines and natural products have been tried to improve nonspecific immunity in cancer patient, which can indirectly help the fight against cancer.

Dr. William Coley, a surgeon from Memorial Cancer Hospital in New York in 1920s, developed a vaccine from mixture of some germs, to be given to cancer patients. He reasoned that such vaccination would challenge the body to fight infections and indirectly would help fight against cancer. This was called as Coley's Toxin and was shown to cause regression of cancer in many patients. This vaccine, when injected, produced acute chills, fever and symptoms of infection for a day or two. Soon the patient would recover from the infection and eventually cancer would regress. Coley reported cancer cure in 41% of patients treated with his vaccine. Unfortunately, Coley's Toxin is no longer available commercially and is not used in conventional cancer treatment.

BCG vaccine is mixture of weakened tuberculosis germs used to immunize against TB. For urinary bladder cancer, when introduced locally, it causes acute bladder infection followed by regression of cancer in some patients. This is an example of nonspecific immunotherapy. Other scientists have developed non-specific vaccines from bacteria and fungi.

Some doctors develop vaccine from patient's own tumor cells, blood cells etc. and re-inject this back into the patient. Many claims have been made for efficacy of such vaccines. However, such vaccine facilities are not widely available. These are practiced mostly by medical centers that deal with alternative medical treatments.

Interferon:

Interferon is a natural protein produced by cells in response to some viruses and foreign substances. It is part of defense mechanism. Interferon can also be produced synthetically by genetic engineering. Interferon alpha is used in certain types of leukemia. The results are variable. It is a type of immunotherapy.

Conclusion:

This chapter has described various conventional treatments for cancer used by modern medicine. Surgery, radiotherapy and chemotherapy are the mainstay of conventional cancer treatments used in modern hospitals. These treatments are aimed at removing or reducing tumor mass. These therapies do not address the root causes of cancer, which is disturbance in the internal condition of body. In spite of successful initial removal of tumor, recurrences are therefore common. Immunotherapy, although ideal for dealing with cancer, has not advanced adequately to be the primary treatment of cancer. A cancer patient and his relatives should discuss all possible benefits and risks of any cancer treatment before undergoing any treatments.

Chapter 9

Treatment: Complementary Alternative Medicine for Cancer

Previous three chapters described the Core, the Foundation and the Conventional treatments of cancer. In this chapter we will review some alternative methods for cancer treatment practiced by some holistic doctors in various centers around the world. The aim of this chapter is to acquaint the reader with what is happening in the different parts of the world in this matter. In writing this chapter, I have extensively used references from the following two books: 1. OPTIONS- The Alternative Cancer Therapy Book by Richard Walters and 2.CANCER: Alternative Medicine Definitive Guide to Cancer by Burton Goldberg, W. John Diamond and W. Lee Cowden.

I neither claim particular results with any such treatments nor recommend any particular treatment. Person interested in knowing more can easily get further information about such methods on the Internet. Finally, your decision to follow any of the following treatment should be taken with discussion with your personal doctors.

This chapter does not include all the different alternative medical methods and undoubtedly there are many more treatment methods reported to have good results. It is important to note that the attention to the core and the foundation, described in earlier chapters, is extremely important not only for complementary treatment of cancer but also for cancer prevention and prevention of many other chronic diseases.

Many of the therapies described below are based on common overlapping concepts. Nutrition and detoxification form the basis for most of such treatments. Use of natural foods, herbs, immune enhancement, detoxification strategies, exercise etc is the common thread running through various complementary and alternative treatments.

AYURVED & HOMEOPATHY:

Ayurved and Homeopathy are two widely practiced medical sciences in India, which will be described in more details in later chapters. Ayurved is the medical science that originated in India. I have personal exposure to these two methods since we have conducted some clinical trials pertaining to Ayurved and Homeopathy over the past few years.

TIBETAN MEDICINE:

Tibetan Medicine is becoming popular in India and abroad. A Himalayan nation north of India, Tibet has close ties with Indian sciences in spirituality, psychology, religion and medicine. Tibetan Medicine is an ancient medical science practiced for many thousand years and has a deep impact from Ayurved. Similar to Ayurved, Tibetan Medicine stresses the importance of 5 elements and 3 dosha, which it names as Wind (Vata), Bile (Pitta) and Phlegm (Kapha). It assumes that all the diseases have a significant mind-body connection. It emphasizes meditation, pranayama and yoga for mental control. Life style changes and good dietary habits are most important part in prevention and treatment of any disease. Like Ayurved, diagnosis of a disease is based on history taking and clinical examination, which includes examination of urine, pulse, tongue, skin etc.

If changes in life style and diet do not adequately help, herbal treatments are considered as the next step. There are various formulas each containing from 3 to 150 Himalayan herbs. These medicines are given orally in tablet forms two or three times a day. In the morning *"Bedken"* type of formula is given mainly for digestive function. At noon time, *"Tripa"* type formula is taken. In the late afternoon or evening, *"Lung"* formulae are used. I think these three types are used sequentially for balancing Kapha: (Phlegm), Pitta: (Bile) and Vata:

(Wind). The patient is examined periodically and formulae are changed as needed.

Many cancer patients have reported good improvements in their condition by using Tibetan Medicine. In India, there are some practitioners of Tibetan Medicine in some big cities. The headquarters are at Mcleod Gunj, Dharamshala in Himachal Pradesh in North India. Dr.Yeshi Dhonden is one of the leading exponents of Tibetan medicine at Dharamshala. For more information, readers may log on to www.tibetanmedicine.com on the Internet or write to Dr. Yeshi Dhonden, Tibetan Herbal Clinic, Mcleod Gunj, Dharamshala, HP, 176219, Phone: 01892-21461. Email: lotsundu@hotmail.com

WHEATGRASS THERAPY:

Many people are familiar with this treatment, which is easy to do at home. Many patients, learning about this from other sources, have started practicing this at their home. Wheatgrass is fresh germinated tender grass grown from wheat. Wheatgrass can be grown in your own house in a series of seven small containers with adequate attention to soil, water and sunlight. The grass has to be consumed raw or in the form of fresh juice around the 7th day. A person can plant small quantity of wheat in a new pot daily over the seven days. After the wheatgrass is taken out from the first pot on the 7th day, the same pot can be used for the next cycle of plantation of wheat seeds. Thus the seven pots used in the first week could be used repeatedly for each weekly cycle of plantation.

Wheatgrass is called a "Live Food". It is a storehouse of chlorophyll and enzymes essential for cell respiration. It is a rich source of vitamin C. It is a natural source of over 100 vitamins, minerals and other nutrients for cells. It has all the essential amino acids, polypeptides and bioflavonoids, which are essential for proper growth and immunity. Sprouted wheat is a rich source of vitamin E. Wheat germs and sprouted wheat seeds have been in common use in India over many centuries to prepare shira, kheer, pudding etc. Wheatgrass has a special

religious significance at the time of harvest and Navaratri-Dasara festivals in India
.

Ann Wigmore developed protocols for wheatgrass therapy. Many holistic doctors are practicing it at various medical centers. This nontoxic therapy combines use of wheatgrass juice with other organically grown raw foods, fresh vegetables, sprouted beans, fruits and nuts. Exercise, mind-body medical methods to uplift mind and cultivation of positive attitude are other key elements in this therapy.

Wheatgrass therapy has been found useful in a wide range of acute and chronic diseases. In treating cancer, the aim is to rebuild the body by providing essential natural nutrients to the cells. These nutrients help body to detoxify the accumulated toxins and waste products. This leads to better immunity against all the diseases. Interested reader is advised to get more information on this subject in various books or on the Internet.

MACROBIOTICS:

Biotic means biological products. Probiotics promote life while antibiotics are supposed to be against (bacterial) life. Macrobiotics is a nutritional system advocating use of special natural foods to fight diseases and promote health. As per Michio Kushi, a leader in macrobiotics movement, "Cancer is a disorder of the body's cells that results largely from improper diet." The concepts of macrobiotics is based on Eastern wisdom with its understanding of complementary forces yin and yang embodying the universal energy principle.

Offering a commonsense alternative to the typical high-fat, low-fiber Western diet associated with cancer and heart disease, macrobiotic diet consists of 50 to 60 percent whole cereal grains; 25 to 30 percent fresh vegetables, smaller amounts of fruits, soups, beans, nuts, sea vegetables and occasional condiments. Chemically treated, highly salted and highly processed foods should be avoided. Daily consumption of Miso soup, made from fermented soybeans, cereal grains and sea salt, has been reported to reduce frequency of stomach cancer as per a medical trial conducted in Japan. Shiitake mushrooms, used in a variety of macrobiotic dishes have powerful anti-tumor effect in mice. Thousands of cancer patients on macrobiotics have reported benefit after strictly following this diet for long periods. Many others, however, did not get any benefit. Patients who are benefited are advised to follow this type of diet for long time even after cancer control.

MOERMAN'S ANTI-CANCER DIET:

Cornelius Moerman (1893-1988), a Dutch physician, helped thousands of cancer patients with his particular diet plans. This therapy is apparently popular in Netherlands and some other European nations. Moerman believed that every cell in the body contains a latent virus capable of developing cancer only when metabolism is disturbed. To put it simply, faulty metabolism triggered by faulty eating is the fundamental cause of cancer.

Antoine Bechamp in France and Guenther Enderlein in Germany demonstrated the existence of a harmless virus normally living in all the cells. Royal Rife and Virginia Livingston, in 20th century, confirmed the presence of such virus (germs) in cells. Later on in this chapter, we will discuss about germ theory of cancer and novel treatment approaches based on this discovery.

The Moerman regimen uses sound nutrition in attempting to reverse the disease process. This immune enhancing approach could help not only cancer patients but also many others afflicted with chronic diseases. Moerman therapy consists of meatless, high-fiber diet rich in vitamins and minerals plus eight supplements found essential for good health: citric acid, iodine, sulfur, vitamins A, B-Complex, C and E. Red beet juice with added vitamin C is also taken to detoxify the blood, especially during and after radiotherapy and chemotherapy treatments. This has been found to greatly reduce the toxic reactions associated with radiotherapy and chemotherapy treatments.

GERSON THERPAY:

Max Gerson, a German physician who immigrated to USA in 1930s, experimented and developed a special approach to chronic diseases. This is known as Gerson Therapy, which has attracted the attention of many physicians round the world. Gerson found his approach very useful to deal with migraine, arthritis, TB, skin diseases and even with cancer. Dr. Gerson thought that restoration of oxygen utilization by the body was the key to deal with chronic diseases. He emphasized on three factors: firstly detoxify body; secondly, fortify body with micronutrients and minerals and lastly, introduce oxidizing enzymes till the body starts making it's own supply of digestive enzymes. This treatment starts with large amounts of vegetable and fruit juices. Cleansing enema with herbs and coffee are given periodically to detoxify the body. Other specific micronutrients and herbs are administered at appropriate time schedule. There are a many cancer patients to testify to the benefits of this approach, which has been so far resisted by the mainstream medicine.

This type of therapy is offered at many centers in Europe, USA and especially in Mexico. Gerson legacy is kept alive by his daughter Charlotte, who runs Gerson International Medical Institute in Tijuana, Mexico. I was fortunate to have met Charlotte Gerson in 1996 in Tijuana to observe the work on cancer patients.

METABOLIC THERAPIES:
A variety of metabolic therapies are in use in various holistic medical clinics around the world. Tijuana, Mexico, a Mexican city just south of the California, is the hub for such medical centers dealing with cancer and other chronic diseases. There are many other places in Europe, Australia, New Zealand, Japan and other parts of the world practicing holistic approach. Metabolic therapy is a multifaceted healing program addressing divergent factors leading to cancer. It uses detoxification to flush out toxins from body. Anti-cancer diets with natural organically grown foods are strictly followed. High doses of vitamins and minerals are given to improve cell function. Proteolytic (protein-breaking)

enzymes make cancer cells easily destroyed by immune cells. These enzymes are known to break down the protein covering of cancer cells, which protects them from destruction from body's immunity. Once this protein coat (kavach in Sanskrit), is broken, cancer cells can be easily attacked, captured and destroyed by body's immune force viz. white blood cells, natural killer cells, interleukins, macrophages etc.

Many enzymes are commercially available as oral supplements. Interestingly, pineapple contains large amounts of bromelain, a source of proteolytic enzymes found useful in cancer. Pineapple forms a part of daily diet in Eastern countries especially Malaysia and Singapore. This tropical fruit is readily available in most parts of the world. You may include pineapple in your diet whenever possible.

Amygdalin, also called as Laetrile, is termed as vitamin B-17. It is a type of carbohydrate occurring naturally in plants e.g. chick-peas (graham-chana- harbara), lentils, lima beans, moong-bean sprouts, cashews, brown rice, wheatgrass etc. Amygdalin is present in the seeds of most of the common fruits. Amygdalin is abundant in dry fruits especially in apricots and almonds. Commercially, amygdalin is produced from kernels of apricot, peaches and bitter almonds. Records show that ancient physicians from China, Greece, Roman Empire and Arabia used these dry fruits (source of amygdalin) for treating various diseases. A recent European trial has shown signs of cancer regression in about 50 percent of cancer patients using amygdalin in metabolic therapies. Including small quantities of dry fruits in your daily diet might be helpful for cancer prevention. Dr. Ernesto Contreras has a large hospital in Tijuana, Mexico, where Amygdalin is used extensively in addition to other complementary therapies for cancer.

Megavitamin therapy, especially high doses of vitamin C, is part of metabolic therapies. Well-known studies by Dr. Linus Pauling, the Nobel Prize winning chemist, and his collaborator Dr Ewan Cameron, showed that large doses of vitamin C markedly improved cancer patient's survival times. Vitamin C, a powerful antioxidant, is known to help in various acute as well as chronic medical conditions. This multipurpose vitamin stimulates immunity and detoxifies the tissues. Vitamin C is naturally plentiful in citrus fruits: lemon, oranges, apples, lime etc. You may include such fruits in your daily diet.

Vitamin, A, E and minerals like selenium, zinc, copper and other trace elements are part of metabolic therapies. This multifaceted approach helps body to detoxify, cells to regenerate and immune function to enhance. This is how metabolic therapy helps as a complementary treatment in cancer.

KELLEY'S THERAPY:

Dr. William Kelley, a physician from Kansas, USA, developed a complex approach to treat many chronic and degenerative diseases including cancer. The three main elements of his nutritional program are nutrition, detoxification and enzyme therapy. He was a controversial figure in the mainstream medical practice but thousands of severely ill patients followed his treatment and reported good results. As per Dr. Kelley, a person gets cancer mainly because he is unable to metabolize the proteins properly in the diet. Instead, the unused proteins are used for tumor growth. That is also the reason why cancer comes back even after apparently successful initial treatment, if the protein metabolism is not corrected. Dr. Kelley linked faulty protein metabolism to a deficiency of pancreatic enzymes, which are responsible for protein digestion. Imbalance of minerals metabolism further interferes with protein digestion making the matters even worse. Additionally, cancer cells produce immune blocking substances to evade the immune surveillance. Kelley's program divides the patients into 10 different metabolic classes, with slow-oxidizing vegetarians on one end and fast-oxidizing meat eaters on the other. Nutritional program is developed individually for different metabolic types. In general, the program recommends consumption of raw organic foods, fruits and vegetables, while protein intake is reduced considerably to preserve the enzymes to digest the fruits and vegetables. Heavy doses of pancreatic enzymes, vitamins, minerals, hormones and some extracts derived from animal organs are administered simultaneously. The regimen also emphasizes various detoxification strategies. Additionally, psychological, mind-body and spiritual support therapies are used. Kelley's therapy is rigorous and not easy to follow for a common person.

NIEPER THERAPY:

A prominent practitioner of holistic medicine in Germany, Dr. Hans Nieper developed a complex nutritional- metabolic therapy for cancer and other chronic diseases. The components of this therapy include correction of mineral imbalance, use of enzymes to dissolve the mucous-protein coat around cancer cells to expose them and gene-repair therapy with some natural substances. Dr. Nieper calls his therapy as " Eumetabolic Therapy". He prescribes varying combinations of vitamins, minerals, amygdalin, animal and plant extracts, pharmaceutical drugs and vaccines for immune stimulation.

HERBS   FOR   CANCER:

Various herbs have been tried, individually or collectively, to treat cancer in various parts of the world at various times. Following is a list of some of the herbs reported to reduce cancer tumor. We do not know if the herbs have a direct anti-cancer activity or these work indirectly through immune stimulation and metabolic improvement. The list is not comprehensive and there could be many other herbs reported to have anti-cancer effect. Before trying any of the following herbal preparations on your own, you must consult a doctor or herbologist to avoid any complications of such treatments.

1. **Algae (Chlorella, sea vegetables, spirulina, green concentrates):** These sea products contain high concentrations of essential proteins, vitamins and minerals. Chlorella, commonly used in Japan, is now being made available in other parts of the world. Spirulina is now available in capsule and powder forms.

2. **Aloe Vera: (Kumari, Koraphad)** is a short plant with thick green leaves, which contain a thick mucoid juice. Ayurved has used this herb extensively over many centuries and found it useful to balance liver metabolism, improve digestion and circulation. It is immune stimulant and helps detoxification. Recently in the West, this herb has attracted attention of medical researchers who have confirmed various health benefits of this herb. It has been found effective in burns, cuts and skin conditions. Aloe emodin, an extract derived from a particular type of aloe seeds, has been reported to have significant activity against leukemia.

3. **Amygdalin, (Laetrile)** present in seeds of many fruits and vegetables. Labeled as Vitamin B-17, this substance is known to enhance immunity and improve metabolism. Abundantly present in kernels of bitter almonds, apricots and peaches.

4. **Astragalus**: An herb used extensively in traditional Chinese Medicine (TCM), astragalus is undergoing extensive clinical trials. One such trial in Japan suggests that a ginseng-astragalus combination may have regulatory effects on NK- Natural Killer cells, an important component of immune system to check cancer. In China, doctors often combine astragalus with another herb called ligustrum. These two mutually enhance individual immune stimulatory properties.

5. **Bhallatak: (Bilawa, Bibwa, Dhobi nut)** *semicarpus anacardium*, a black nut found mostly in India, Bhallatak has been used in Ayurveda over many centuries. Dr. B. G. Wad from Mumbai, who reported it's anti-cancer properties, extensively tested the extracts of this nut. Based on his research, a local pharmaceutical company in Mumbai developed Anacarcin, a product containing extracts of Bhallatak. The raw juice from this nut is highly allergenic and needs to be processed in a specific way for medicinal use. Dr. B. N. Purandare, another prominent medical doctor from Mumbai, used Bhallatak to treat

several of his female patients suffering from cancer of uterus. I had personal discussions with Dr. Wad and Dr. Purandare about utility of this herb in cancer treatment. Dr. Wad discovered low-level radioactivity emanating from fresh extracts of this nut.

I have used this substance in combination with other conventional treatments on several of my cancer patients. I found that this addition usually helped to improve the disease free survival in majority of patients. Dr. A. V. Bavadekar, a leading orthopedic surgeon from Mumbai, himself used Bhallatak in addition to other treatments for his own gastric cancer, which has been now in complete remission for more than 12 years. Dr. Bavadekar has given detailed account about his successful personal fight against cancer in his Marathi book " *Cancer Maza Sangati*" (meaning My Companion Cancer).

For personal use, broken bhallatak nuts have to be boiled in milk to make a decoction, which can be consumed in small quantities. You need precise guidance to use Bhallatak, which is a toxic and allergenic product. It does not suit everyone. An Ayurvedic physician may be able to analyze your constitution and instruct you on the proper use of this product.

6. **Cat's Claw: (*Unacaria tomentosa*)** This is a herb from South American rain forests, traditionally used as a tribal medicine for arthritis, cancer and many other diseases. It is an immune enhancing, antioxidant digestion-promoting herb. It contains several types of antioxidants: polyphenols, triterpines and plant steroids. It has been reported to help in brain tumors and other types of cancers.

7. **Echinacea:** A common herb used in Europe and USA, echinacea is used primarily to fight acute infections, colds etc. It has been used in complementary fashion to boost immunity through stimulation of NK cell activity in cancer patients.

8. **Essiac:** This is a mixture of herbs originally known to Native American Indians in Ontario, Canada. In 1920s, a Canadian nurse named Rene Caisse came across these herbs being used on a breast cancer a tribal woman. Caisse experimented with this formula and confirmed its benefits. It was developed as an herbal tea and named Essiac, (which is caisse spelt backwards)! Caisse and her associates recorded many impressive case histories attesting to its efficacy in cancer.

9. **Flavonoids:** This is class of natural substances derived from bright colored fruits and vegetables. Flavonoids are some of the best-known natural substances to fight cancer. These are present in tomatoes, carrots, beets, grape, apples and many other citrus fruits and vegetables. Grape seeds are a rich source of Bioflavonoids. Unfortunately, with the development of seedless grapes, it is now hard to find grapes with seeds for eating! Flavonoids are free radical scavengers that remove toxins and waste products from tissues. These are an important part of nutrition to fight cancer.

10. **Garlic:** A household herb in cooking, garlic has shown many medicinal uses. Scientific research in Japan, China and Italy has suggested that regular consumption of garlic can reduce the risk of stomach cancer by about 50%. Animal studies have shown that aged garlic extract appears to stop the growth of cancers of breast, bladder, skin and colon. It also reduces the risk of cancers of esophagus, stomach and lungs. Garlic helps to relieve the side effects of radiation and chemotherapy such as loss of appetite and fatigue. Garlic protects DNA from damage from carcinogens. The First World Congress on Health Significance of Garlic held recently concluded, " Garlic in various forms; from cooked garlic, garlic oil, raw garlic juice, garlic powder and aged garlic extract, can provide health benefits of reducing heart disease and cancer risk". One word of caution: According to Ayurveda, garlic may not suit to persons of Pitta constitution. You have to experiment yourself whether or not garlic suits you.

11. **Gingko Biloba:** A Chinese medicinal herb used for thousands of years has antioxidant properties to remove free radical toxins from body. It reduces the free radical damage and improves immunity. Gingko is also reported to reduce platelet-activating factor in the blood, PAF, which is suspected to promote cancer process.

12. **Ginger:** Ginger is a common household herb. It does have a complementary role in health maintenance. Ginger restores disturbed digestive functions. It stimulates *Agni,* which in Sanskrit means fire. In the external world, fire cooks the food and burns up the dross. In the body, agni is responsible for proper digestion in stomach and for assimilation of various nutrients in all the tissues. When agni is strong, toxic waste products in the body are disposed properly. When the appetite is poor, ginger can help. Shredded fresh ginger mixed with equal parts of fresh lemon juice and pure honey should be prepared daily. A teaspoon of this mixture can be eaten before mealtime to stimulate appetite and help digestion. This formula also works to reduce the nausea and vomiting associated with chemotherapy and radiotherapy treatments. In episodes of diarrhea, dysentery and gastro-enteritis, this simple household formula has been found to be effective. Lemon juice contains natural vitamin C, which acts as an antioxidant. Honey helps in digestion and provides important natural sugars and minerals.

13. **Ginseng (Panax):** This herb has been in use in China for more than 2000 years. It is used for strength, vitality, emotional stability and wisdom! The Chinese variety is different from Siberian Ginseng. Recent research on Ginseng has identified many active ingredients including saponins, essential oils, phytosterols, amino acids, peptides, vitamins and minerals. Saponins have been shown to stimulate NK cell and macrophage activity, an important part of immunity. Ginseng acts as a free radical scavenger. Korean research has

demonstrated that regular use of ginseng can reduce cancer risk more than 50 %. Ginseng is termed as an Adaptogen- helping body to adapt to stressful situation. Ashwagandha, an Indian herb used in Ayurved to increase strength and vitality, is sometimes called Indian Ginseng, although it is not related to Panax Ginseng.

14. **Grape Seed Extract:** There are a number of health benefits in grapes and their seeds. There are anecdotal reports of cancers being cured by eating only grapes for few months. We do not know if eating grapes alone in place of regular food is a right nutritional approach. Grape seeds are a rich source of pychnogenols, bioflavonoids and anthrocyanins, phytochemicals known to help immunity and detoxification. Grape seed extracts can help in many other chronic degenerative diseases. In the West, grape seed extracts are available in capsule forms in health food stores and drug stores. With development of seedless grape technology, grape seeds have disappeared from the market. However, it might be advisable to eat whole old-fashioned grapes with seeds, if one can get. It is claimed that grape seeds can 1. Improve blood and lymph circulation, 2. Reduce thickening of arteries thus reducing risk of heart disease, 3. Improve eyesight and skin health, 4. Protect brain, nerves and memory, and 5. Help function of muscles and joints.

15. **Green Tea:** Large amount of green tea are consumed daily by Chinese and Japanese. Recent research shows that green tea is a rich source of Catechins, cancer fighting plant chemicals. Catechins are even more effective than vitamin E in defending body against free radicals. Studies have shown that regular consumption of green tea can reduce risk of cancers of liver, esophagus, colon and bladder. Green tea, black tea and oolong tea are the three types of tea that are produced by different processes on fresh tea leaves.

16. **Soybeans:** Originated in the Far East, soybeans are now available worldwide. There are proponents as well as opponents for use of soybean products. Soybeans are a rich source of zinc, selenium, vitamins A, B1, B2, B12, C, D and K, as well as many amino acids. It is recommended that only soybeans grown organically without any chemical fertilizers should be used after adequate fermentation to get health benefits. Fermentation splits soy proteins into amino acids and liberates phytosterols, saponins and isoflavons. These nutrients are all important in cancer prevention.

17. **Hansi:** Dr. Hirschmann, an Argentinean biologist, developed homeopathically prepared combinations of rain forest herbs. Hansi stands for Homeopathic Activator of Natural System of Immunity. Hansi is also childhood nickname of Dr Hirschmann. It is a combination of low potency (3X to 11X) extracts from aloe, cactus, arnica, lachesis, lycopodium and other natural substances customized to different disease conditions. Hansi is available in liquid form as well as for injections. At present, Hansi is legally available as a drug in Mexico, Argentina, Bahamas and Hungary. These combinations probably enhance functions of liver, spleen, kidney, lungs, bowel and skin that are responsible for detoxification. Hansi supplies micronutrients in homeopathic dosages.

18. **Hoxsey Herbs:** Harry Hoxsey was a doctor who developed an herbal therapy practiced by his grand father in Illinois, USA. The elder Hoxsey witnessed his horse, suffering from terminal cancer, getting cured by grazing on certain plants. The plants were studied and Hoxsey family developed a formula of herbs, for external application as well as internal use. Harry Hoxsey attracted thousands of cancer patients from all over USA, many of whom seem to get better. Cancers that have responded favorably include lymphoma, melanoma and skin cancer. The classic Hoxsey formula comes in potassium iodide solution and contains red clover, buckthorn bark, burdock root, stillingia root,

barberry bark, chaparral, licorice root, cascara amarga, and prickly ash bark. Hoxsey met with a lot of resistance from medical establishment for his promotion of this herbal treatment. Today, Hoxsey treatment is being offered for cancer at Bio-Medical Center in Tijuana, Mexico.

19. **Iscador (Mistletoe):** Mistletoe is a shrub growing in parasitic form on various other trees. Iscador is made from mistletoe, which are shrubs growing as parasites on other trees. Similarly, cancer tumor grows on body as a parasite. Mistletoe had been held sacred by ancient Celts and Germans and often credited with medicinal properties. European doctors are using Iscador since 1920s.There are different varieties of Iscador recommended for different tumor types. Therapeutic benefits have been reported in over 5000 medical studies world over. Iscador is given as a series of injections, two or three times weekly. It stimulates immunity as evidenced by increase in number of NK cells, macrophages and inhibits cancer growth. In India, many homeopathic and alternative medical practitioners make Iscador treatment available.

20. **Medicinal Mushroom:** Japanese traditions cherish searching for wild forest mushrooms, which have been claimed to have miraculous healing powers. According to researchers at the National Cancer Center in Japan, complete tumor elimination was seen in experimentally induced cancers in animals, which were fed with extracts from maitake, shiitake and reishi mushrooms. These three are the main varieties of mushroom used for medicinal properties. Currently, such mushrooms are cultivated in mushroom farms for commercial supply. Mushroom extract exhibits anti-cancer activity inhibiting carcinogenesis and metastases. It enhances immune functions. Germanium, a trace element found in organic form in mushroom, is reported to improve oxygen consumption by body tissues. Cancer cells are unable to grow in the presence of adequate oxygen within tissue.

21. **Pau-D-Arco:** The herbal extract from the bark of Pau-D-Arco tree found in the South American rain forests offers another option in cancer treatment. The main active ingredient is called lapachol, which has shown a strong anti-cancer action. Lapachol can be taken in capsule form or as an herbal tea made out of Pau-D-Arco, which is freely available at many health food stores in USA and Europe.

22. **Ranavila:** In 1980s, Dr. Ramesh Dhokte, an Ayurvedic doctor from Bombay, studied a tribal herb growing in the western hills of India. As the story goes, a tribal medicine woman introduced Dr Dhokte to this herb from Mahabaleshwar, a hilly resort in the state of Maharashtra. Dr. Dhokte experimented and developed a treatment plan combining Ranavila with other Ayurvedic medicines plus strict dietary plans. Varying degrees of success rates have been claimed for his treatment method.

23. **Sarvapishti:** Dr.Trivedi, an Ayurvedic researcher from Varanasi, India, developed a white powder from hundreds of edible plants and herbs. This powder, being taken as a daily nutritional supplement, has reportedly helped thousands of cancer patients in India and abroad. New York based oncologist Dr. Suhrid Parekh recently testified, in a local Bombay newspaper, that his pancreatic cancer was in remission due to daily consumption of Sarvapishti. The pancreatic cancer, which was growing in spite of three cycles of chemotherapy taken earlier, had shown significant shrinkage with Sarvapishti. A book of 110 case studies on cancer patients treated with Sarvapishti was recently published in India. Some cancer specialists in Bombay suggested that a placebo controlled clinical trial should have been undertaken to confirm the benefits. Such trials are difficult to perform without the cooperation of modern cancer hospitals. There are many difficult ethical and moral issues in such trials. Some proponents of herbal medicines argue that randomized placebo-

controlled double blind trials have not even been conducted on most of the chemotherapy drugs, which are in common use these days. These scientists wonder why different yardstick should be applied to herbal medicines, which have been found to be useful by many cancer patients. It might be interesting to perform double blind trials on patients receiving oral chemotherapy capsules on one hand and herbal capsules on the other hand.

24. **Turmeric (Haladi):** Turmeric, a bright yellow spice belonging to ginger family, is used extensively in Indian cooking. In Ayurved, turmeric is known for its' anti-septic, anti-inflammatory and digestive properties. Recent research indicates that turmeric can inhibit cancer at various stages of development. In one study, turmeric was shown to decrease the formation of abnormal DNA after exposure to benzoapyrene, a cancer-causing chemical. This suggests anti-cancer, anti-oxidant and immunity enhancing properties of turmeric. The main active component of turmeric is called curcumin. Turmeric combined with betel leaf was found to be more effective against oral cancer than when either ingredient was used alone. For a long time, betel leaf and betel nut have been blamed for high incidence of oral cancer in India. Time has come to review whether the betel leaf is the real culprit or if there are other reasons such as poor oral hygiene, tooth infections and injuries from sharp teeth for cancer promotion. Ayurved recommends use of betel leaf to promote digestion and as a medicine for certain conditions.

25.

AUTO-URINE THERAPY,
SHIVAMBU CHIKITSA:

This is a controversial subject. I do not personally recommend auto-urine therapy for my patients. From time to time, some patients ask me whether they should take urine therapy. The idea of drinking urine, which is excreted as a waste product by the body, is repulsive. However, I have seen patients, willingly undertaking such a task, at ease with this method. Some of these patients even reported to be improving under this treatment! I leave the choice to each patient.

The details of the urine therapy are mentioned in some ancient Indian books. Ayurved stresses use of cow's urine for preparation of many medicines. Dr. Dadasaheb Bhoge, a senior Ayurvedic practitioner in Grant Road, Mumbai, was a staunch proponent of urine therapy. I had met him a few times and he always discussed the benefits of auto-urine therapy- shivambu. (In Sanskrit, *Shiva*= Lord Shiva also meaning inner Self, and *Ambu* = water). Thus, *shivambu* means own urine. Dr. Bhoge wrote several articles and books on this subject. Former Prime Minister of India, Mr. Morarji Desai was a strong supporter of this method.

Alternative medicine highlights the importance of detoxification, which means removing the toxic waste products from the body. Kidney is an important organ to get rid of dissolved toxic waste products from the body. Logically speaking, drinking urine would defeat the purpose of detoxification.

While searching articles, I came across a few points, which might explain why auto-urine therapy might be working. Urea is a natural end-product of protein digestion in the body. About 30 grams of urea, which gives the particular stench to urine, is daily excreted in the urine. Urea has been used as a medicine since 1940s. Dr. Danopoulos, a noted Greek physician, reported substantial benefits from using urea in liver cancer. When given orally, urea reaches highest concentrations in the liver and inhibits cancer growth. Urea appears to dissolve the fibrin stroma (protein matrix around cells) and inhibits the formation of new blood vessels in tumor. This may be one explanation how it works in cancer. Liver is the only organ where urea is concentrated, after which it is excreted in urine. Therefore it is suggested that urea would help treat only liver cancers. Dr. Danopoulos found that injections of urea directly into the tumor mass also helped shrink the cancers.

In 1960s, Dr. Stanislaw Burzinski from Texas isolated some peptides (amino acid chains) from human urine and found them effective in controlling growth of certain cancers. He found these peptide molecules work on tumor suppressor genes and thus switch off the growth signal for cancer cells. Dr. Burzinski termed these peptides as Antineoplastons, anti= against, neoplastones= new growth= cancer. He developed different protocols for different tumors. Animal studies in Japan indicate that low doses of synthetic antineoplaston- A10 help prevent cancers of breast, lung and liver.
Whether or not to use auto-urine therapy is a personal decision to be taken by the patient. There are many books in English and local languages in India which provide details of this method. I have no personal recommendation, either for or against auto-urine therapy.

CARTILAGE THERAPY:

Cartilage is a special soft elastic tissue from which bones are formed. Cartilage is present in ears, in the septum of nose and at the growing ends of bones in children. Dr. William Lane, PhD, found that cartilage of shark had anticancer properties. He published a book "Why Sharks Don't Get Cancer", which became very popular. In 1970s, researchers at the Massachusetts Institute of Technology found that injections of shark cartilage stopped tumor growth in laboratory animals within 20 days. Other workers have reported encouraging results. The subject is still controversial and opposed by the mainstream cancer doctors. Shark cartilage has now become a big industry in the West.

In 1954, John Prudden M.D. discovered that Bovine Tracheal Cartilage, BTC, had remarkable ability to heal the wounds. It works through supply of healthy cells of cartilage to the healing wounds in patients. Dr. Prudden further found that BTC also had some anticancer properties. BTC decreases the formation of new blood vessels in tumor, thereby causing tumor shrinkage. It also stimulates immune function. In one study, BTC was shown to be effective as a complementary treatment in patients of cancers of ovary, pancreas, colon and testis.

Some people may have reservations about using this animal product on ethical ground. Bovine cartilage is much more readily available than the shark cartilage. Cartilage treatment is not a cure for cancer; it is only a supplemental treatment. Patients opting for this have to continue taking large doses of cartilage for lifetime for continued effect, which may be another drawback.

DMSO:
This natural substance, Di- Methyl- Sulfur- Oxide, is present in minute quantities in many grains, fruits and vegetables. It is organic chemical solvent that can also be derived from coal, oils and some plant lignans. DMSO is present in very small quantities in some tissues. In medicine, especially in veterinary medicine, it is used locally to reduce inflammation. DMSO acts on cell walls and alters the permeability, thereby accelerating process of throwing out the toxins in cells as well as helping absorption of nutrients into cells. In cancer, it is shown to induce cellular differentiation, the process by which aggressive cancer cells become less malignant. DMSO stimulates various parts of immune system and also scavenges free hydroxyl radicals. DMSO, when used simultaneously with chemotherapy, was shown to increase effect of chemotherapy. It might help reduce the dosage of chemotherapy drugs without reducing their effect on cancer. DMSO can be given by injections or even by mouth in a liquid form. It can also be applied as an ointment on cancer tumors. Due to its' Sulfur contents, DMSO gives a peculiar garlic like smell to the person consuming this chemical. It has to be used under proper medical supervision.

GLUTATHIONE & NAC (n- acetyl cystein):

Glutathione is a protein consisting of amino acids cystein, glycine and Glutamic acid. These amino acids are very important for liver function and for removing toxins from body tissues. N- acetyl cystein is used as an injection in cases of poisoning due to overdose of certain pharmaceutical drugs. Glutathione and NAC are found to repair damage to DNA and thus play an important complementary role in cancer treatment.

HYDRAZINE SULFATE:

In research trials, this chemical was shown to inhibit loss of proteins and help preserve the weight in cancer patients. It may be of some use when a cancer patient starts loosing weight. It inhibits a liver enzyme thereby decreasing formation of glucose on which cancer cells thrive. It was found effective in partially shrinking cancer tumors in various clinical trials. This medicine is given orally.

COW'S MILK, BUTTER & GHEE:

Ayurved has recommended use of butter and ghee (clarified butter) since ancient times for strength, health and luster. Strangely, support for this concept is now being offered by modern science. Ghee has it's peculiar flavor due to butyric acid, a fatty acid. Butyric acid and its salts are found to convert malignant cancer cells into normal cells. "Cancer Chemotherapy Reports" published in 1975, and "Deutshe Medizinsche Wochenschrift" a German periodical published in 1969 have research articles about beneficial results of butyric acid products in cancer. In the current age of " Low Cholesterol, Fat Free Diets" it would be worthwhile to remember that good fats are essential for good health. I feel that everyone might benefit by daily consumption of moderate quantity of good fats, pure ghee being one example of such fats. Other naturally available essential fatty acids are mentioned elsewhere in this book.

BIOLOGICAL DENTISTRY:

Dental health has a tremendous impact on health and illness of body. European researchers estimate that perhaps as many as 50 % chronic degenerative diseases are linked, directly or indirectly, to dental problems. Chinese medicine states that each tooth is connected by an acupuncture meridian with a different internal organ. Disease of a tooth can lead to disease of an internal organ and conversely, a disease of internal organ can lead to a disease of that particular tooth. . Infected tooth can release some biological toxins leading to chronic ill health.

Modern diet habits have led to epidemic of dental decay and infections. Earlier, mercury-silver amalgams were often used by dentists to fill up the dental cavities. It is reported that such fillings release minute amount of poisonous mercury compounds in circulation. Over the years, toxic effects of mercury can lead to chronic ill health. Biological dentists stress use of non-toxic restoration material for dental work. There is also some controversy about the root canal treatments, which is a common procedure these days. Each tooth has microscopic web of micro channels, which may not be completely sterilized in spite of careful preparations for root canal therapy. In spite of apparently successful root canal therapy, it is claimed by some holistic dental practitioners that micro-level chronic infection persists in the treated tooth. This might be a toxic source of future trouble.

German Physician Dr. Josef Issels, whom I met in Los Angeles in 1996, states " Even after the most precise preparation of the main root canal, proteins will always remain in the tiny interconnecting canals…If proteins become infected, the toxins produced by microbes in a tooth with root filling can no longer be evacuated in the mouth, but…. are conveyed to the tonsils and flow systems of body". This might be a source for chronic illness including cancer. Doctors practicing biological dentistry take all these factors into account before deciding a proper line of dental care.

NATUROPATHY:

Naturopathy is using natural substances and nature's powers for healing. This is a very expansive subject with wide coverage as per the orientations of individual practitioner. In this book, I am trying to give my own views about naturopathy, which are obviously not all-inclusive. Each naturopath might have his own special ways of treating illness. There are many naturopathic centers around the world and you may come across many different naturopathic methods practiced at various places. Naturopathy, used a complementary method, might help restore the natural balance to help the body to overcome a disease. As with any other "pathy", the results of such treatments are variable and cannot be guaranteed. Hindu philosophy and Ayurved state the five basic elements responsible for creation of the universe, Pancha- Mahabhoota, which are Earth, Water, Fire, Air and Space. Application of mud to a diseased part would be putting earth element to medical use. Similarly, protocols for Water Therapy, Heat Therapy, Color-Light Therapy, Magnetic Therapy, and Mantra Therapy have been evolved. People have reported health benefits from bathing in hot water springs at various locations. Water is essential for life and for all the functions of cells. Following is a brief description of some of the treatments using the elements.

WATER THERAPY:
Water therapy, also called as hydrotherapy, uses water in many forms such as hot or cold water, steam, vapor, ice etc. Water can be used externally for bath, sauna, and local applications or can be taken internally. Some doctors recommend drinking 2 to 3 liters of plain pure water daily. People drinking more than 1.5 liters of water daily have reduced risk of developing bladder cancers. Drinking large amount of water on getting up in the morning stimulates the movements of intestines thereby helping the passage of stools naturally. It washes away the toxins and accumulated waste from intestines. Water should be taken as pure plain water. Fruit juices, soft drinks and other liquid foods, which may be consumed as per personal choice, are no substitute for water therapy. If you provide the luxury of plenty of water to the body, body will function better. To give a simile, one can either wipe the floor of the room with wet cloth or scrub the floor with bucketful of

water, which might clean the room much better. The body will be able to remove toxins dissolved in urine better if plenty of water is available. People with kidney problems and swellings should consult their physicians before drinking large amounts of water.

Lack of adequate water in the body may lead to dehydration. Drinking large amounts of water would make blood circulate with ease. The kidneys throw out excess water in urine. Water makes cells to exchange nutrients, wastes and toxins easily across the cell membrane. Water facilitates all the biochemical actions in body. Many chronic health problems such as migraine, high blood pressure, constipation, kidney stones, prostate problems, arthritis, fatigue, circulatory problems etc. have reportedly improved after regular consumption of large amounts of water.

The metabolic work makes body cells somewhat acidic. The term pH, which means potential hydrogen, is a scale to express relative acidity or alkalinity of any substance. The scale extends from 1 to 14, the midpoint reading of 7 is neutral, neither acidic nor alkaline. Distilled water, being totally neutral and free of minerals, has pH of 7. Body mechanisms maintain blood pH strictly between. 7.35 to 7.45. Even if a lot of acid radicals are produced in the body, blood in health is always maintained as slightly alkaline around 7.4 in spite of other tissues becoming more acidic or alkaline. Many diseases including cancer grow rapidly in acidic surroundings. Different foods can increase or decrease the acidity in the body.

Originated in Japan, microwater or micronized water is a new filter system with potential health benefits. Water is separated in two compartments and electric DC current is passed through electrodes submerged in each compartment. After few minutes, due to electrolysis, water in one compartment becomes acidic and other one alkaline. Alkaline water can reduce body acidity if taken as a drink frequently. The acidic water in the other compartment, which kills germs, can be used for cleaning vegetables, utensils and even to clean wounds. Many health conscious people all around the world are now using microwater machines. This is natural way of counteracting acidity in the body. Special foods, some chemicals and medicines can also be taken to decrease the acidity in the body. Testing saliva with a special litmus paper is a simple way to determine the actual pH of body tissues, which may be different than the blood pH and urine pH.

Gold-activated Water Therapy: This is a simple method described by Ayurved to make your everyday drinking water more beneficial for your health. A pure gold article, usually a gold ring or bracelet is hung with a string in the middle of a pot. Pot is filled with water and it is made to boil for about 10 minutes. This water, which is consumed for drinking during the day, has been shown to help detoxification of the body. This simple, inexpensive method can be tried by anyone. Gold is an important noble element used by Ayurved for removing toxins, purification, strength and rejuvenation. The water thus made is supposed to be activated by gold, although no actual gold molecules can be found in such water.

HEAT THERAPY:
There are various methods of applying heat, which cleans the body of germs, toxins and waste products. Holistic doctors look upon fever as a natural reaction to destroy the germs that cause infection. Artificial fever is deliberately induced by some injections to hasten the fight against certain diseases. Josef Issels, a German physician, is pioneer of fever therapy for treating various conditions and cancer with injections that induce fever. Heat has shown many other health benefits. It is an everyday experience that some muscular aches and pains are relieved by application of heat pads or hot water bottles. In steam bath and sauna, heat acts on your skin, causes perspiration that helps detoxification through the skin.

Modern day physiotherapists use diathermy, microwave and infrared machines to treat various diseases by heat. Hyperthermia, which means increase in temperature, is used successfully in treatment of certain cancers. Sophisticated hyperthermia machines, using microwaves or ultrasonic waves are being used alone or in conjunction with radiotherapy treatments for dealing with cancer.

COLOR THERAPY:
Light consists of a spectrum of different colors. Seven colors of the rainbow are well known with their countless shades. Yoga science describes seven chakras in human body; at Crown, Eyebrow, Throat, Heart, Naval, Sacrum and lastly Basal at lower end of spinal column. A chakra acts as an interface, somewhat like a transformer, between cosmic prana energy and individual prana energy within the body. Each chakra is responsible for some specific actions in the body related to circulation of prana in the subtle channels called nadis. Yogis have perceived specific colors related to each chakra. Color therapy, which consists of exposing body part to a specific color of light, claims to restore deficient color vibrations to body to improve health. Sophisticated expensive machines are now being made in Europe and other Western nations and being exported. Real utility of color therapy, however, is controversial and subject to individual experiences.

MAGNETIC THERAPY:
This controversial subject is a topic of hot discussions amongst the proponents and the opponents. There are many individual stories of success in treatment of cancer with magnetic therapy. Some scientific studies have shown that cancer tumor decreased in size after prolonged exposure to negative (North Pole) magnetic field while it increased when exposed to the opposite positive (South Pole) field. Wolfgang Ludwig in Germany, John Zimmerman of Nevada, Dr. William Philpot of Oklahoma and many other scientists in Russia, Europe, USA and Japan have done extensive research on magnetic therapy. Negative side of magnet (North pole), which normalizes metabolism, has a calming and healing effect. The positive South Pole has stressful effect. It is suggested that North Pole side of the magnet should be applied to the cancer bearing area of body. Magnetic therapy should be undertaken under the supervision of a trained magneto-therapist. It is customary to keep the drinking water container above the north pole of a magnet

overnight and then use such "Magnetized Water" during the day for drinking.

VACCINES FOR CANCER TREATMENT:
Since Edward Jenner first discovered small pox vaccine, many researchers have developed vaccines for many infections. Vaccines are prepared from weakened germ cells and toxins known to causes certain diseases. Vaccines offer body's immune cells a chance to organize and fight against those diseases. It is similar to the training in a military camp for future war. Cancer is not an infection in usual sense of the word. Cancer cells are known to carry antigens. Antigens are protein molecules on the surfaces of germs as well as cancer cells, which are recognized as an "Enemy" by immune cells. Antigens evoke reaction from immune cells, which develop antibodies to fight against those antigens.

Non-specific vaccines like BCG have been used to stimulate immunity in the fight against cancer. Cancer Vaccine is a very complex subject and too technical to describe in this book. Many medical centers around the world are experimenting with vaccine therapy and reporting beneficial results in patients. Antigens are isolated either from patient's own tumor, from other patient's tumor or from cancer cell cultures in the laboratory. After special processing, vaccines are made out of this material and injected into cancer patients. This is a type of immunotherapy, which is still under developmental stage. Success rates vary from clinic to clinic.

OXYGEN AND OZONE THERAPY:
Dr. Otto Warburg, Nobel Prize winner from Germany, discovered that lack of oxygen stimulated growth of cancer cells. For many decades, scientists have tried to improve oxygenation of cells by different methods. Fresh air, difficult to access these days, consists of 78% Nitrogen, 21 % Oxygen plus smaller amounts of Carbon dioxide and other rare gases. With proper exercise, deep breathing and normal lungs, a person can usually supply adequate oxygen to blood and body cells. In cancer patients, various additional methods have been

developed to supply extra oxygen. Even if oxygen is given to the patient, the lungs and body cells should be enabled to use this oxygen rich air.

Oxygen can be given through the rubber tubes inserted in the nose. This oxygen rich air will partly improve the oxygen concentration of blood. Blood should have adequate hemoglobin, the iron containing red pigment in the red blood cells, which carries the oxygen from cell to cell. Some patients are kept in plastic tent connected to oxygen supply.

Ozone is a potent form of oxygen. Oxygen molecule has two atoms of oxygen joined together while ozone has three atoms of oxygen. Ozone can give up additional active atom of oxygen readily for any biochemical activity in the cells. Ozone is produced either from atmospheric oxygen or from pure oxygen by passage of high voltage electric currents. Lightening in thunderstorms produces natural ozone in atmosphere. Ozone can be recognized by a peculiar smell during thunderstorms. Similarly, Ozone is produced in the vicinity of engineering workshops where high voltage electric sparks are used for welding. Ozone layer around the Earth absorbs harmful solar radiations thus protecting life on earth. Ozone machines are available for personal and hospital uses. There are various ways of using Ozone.

Like oxygen, ozone can be made to circulate in a plastic tent where a patient sits. Ozone is absorbed through skin as well as through breathing. Ozone is too strong to be given directly through a rubber tube in the nose. Ozone can also be mixed in water, which is used for bathing. Dissolved ozone gets absorbed through the skin during bath. Air mixed with Ozone can be introduced in the colon during an enema. This Ozone, besides removing local toxins and germs in the colon, quickly enters circulation and purifies the blood. This procedure is a part of colonic detoxification. In some clinics, patient's blood is removed in a bottle and Ozone is bubbled through this blood for a few minutes. Dark blackish blood then turns bright red with Ozone. The pure red oxygenated blood is then injected back into the patient. Ozone treatments, in various forms, are reported to help greatly in various infections, chronic diseases and even in cancer patients.

Hydrogen Peroxide: H2O2 is a water molecule with an extra oxygen atom. This liquid in dilute form is used for gargles and for cleaning wounds. The extra oxygen helps to kill the germs and disinfects debris. In some clinics, minute quantities of hydrogen peroxide are added to the intra-venous solutions and given to patients. This method should be used very cautiously since wrong dosage can produce more harm than good.

BIOELECTRIC & BIOLOGICAL THERAPIES BASED ON GERM THEORY OF CANCER:

Cancer is not an infection like typhoid, cholera, pneumonia, tonsillitis etc. Modern medicine states that cancer is not related to a specific germ. Germ Theory of infections, developed by Louise Pasteur in France in 1857, states that a separate germ is responsible for each infectious disease. Cancer does not spread by contact like many other infectious diseases. Specific infections are due to specific germs. However, some very interesting contradictory observations were made on "Germ Theory" by Antoine Bechamp, a contemporary and rival of Pasteur. Bechamp stated that all the living beings always harbour innocent viral like particles in the cells and in the extracellular parts of body. These living particles can be seen only under darkfield microscopy of living tissue. The particles cannot be identified by conventional microscopy, which examines dead tissue after fixing and staining the slides.

Many other workers, especially Guenther Enderlein of Germany, Gaston Naessens of France, Dr. Royal Rife and Dr. Virginia Livingston both from USA, later on confirmed Bechamp's observations. These naturally present innocent living germs were variously termed as Somatids, Protits and Progenitor cryptocides by these workers. It was shown that under unhealthy internal conditions, these innocent germs could change form to become different viruses, bacteria and even fungi and manifest different infective diseases. Further research revealed that many chronic diseases and even cancer are associated with aggressive forms of protits. We have already discussed this matter in more details in earlier chapter on Causes of Cancer.

Livingston Therapy:
Various biological treatments, using injections and oral liquids, to restore the pathogenic germs to original innocent primitive forms were developed in Germany, France and USA. Dr. Livingston developed a treatment protocol, which combined administration of custom made vaccines with nutritional supplements, detoxification, biological dentistry and heat therapy. In 1968, Livingston founded Livingston-Wheeler Medical Clinic in San Diego, California, for treatment of cancer.

Sanum Remedies:
Based on the work of Enderlein, SANUM biological remedies were developed to restore the internal balance and to revert the germs to innocent forms. Sanum remedies are dilutions of bacteria and fungi, which, when given to the patient, reverse the disease process and bring about a cure. There are many reports of successfully treating cancer and other chronic conditions with Sanum remedies.

Rife Electro-therapy:
In 1930s and 1940s, Dr Royal Rife, a doctor and scientist in California, did extensive research on cancer. He developed a special microscope, through which he could repeatedly confirm the presence of harmless protits changing into disease producing germs. Rife observed a particular form of virus, which he termed as BX virus, constantly associated with majority of the cancer tumors. With strenuous research extending over many decades, Rife developed an electrical machine to treat cancer patients. This machine generated radio frequency and audio frequency waves that could be directed to the cancer bearing area of the patients. Dr. Rife found that at a certain critical frequency, these BX cancer viruses get destroyed. Detailed reports are still available showing successful cancer treatment even in many terminal cancer patients treated with Rife Machines. Dr. Rife met with a lot of opposition from

the medical establishment and his research was suppressed. In the last 2 decades, there has been renewed interest in Rife technology, which is being tested and made available. Various versions of Rife Machines are being developed. Some machines apply frequency micro currents directly to the body parts involved with cancer. Other machines emit electromagnetic radiations, which are directed to the patient. Still another versions generate audio-frequency waves to be used for the treatment. It has been claimed that bioelectrical therapies can successfully treat not only cancer but also many other chronic degenerative diseases and even acute infections as well.

CONCLUSION:

The complementary and alternative treatment options are countless. This chapter describes only some of these options. Information about Ayurved and Homeopathy will be given separately in later chapters. The purpose of this chapter is only to inform the reader about some methods practiced by different centers. The author neither recommends any particular treatment nor guarantee any cures. There are undoubtedly many more methods, not listed here, claimed to be effective in cancer treatment. From the periphery of a circle, each radius leads to the center. There are countless radii, each leading to the center of the circle. Similarly, there are many methods of treatment; the common central aim is to cure the disease. If you need to know more about any particular method of treatment, I suggest you log on Internet and search for the specific words. Volumes of information are currently available on World Wide Web, which seems to ever expand incredibly.

Chapter 10

PSYCHOLOGY OF CANCER

Modern medicine is now becoming increasingly aware about the connection between mind and body in health as well as in disease. Symptoms are what a patient expresses about his suffering. Signs are what doctors find on medical examination or by means of medical tests. There may not be a consistent relationship between findings on the reports and patient's perceived suffering. Symptoms may vary greatly for a specific finding on the report. For example, a patient might be experiencing severe chest pains but the chest x-ray and cardiogram may be normal. Conversely, having an abnormal cardiogram and a big spot on chest x-ray, the patient may be without any symptoms. Experience of pain, depression, anxiety, fear etc is mostly subjective feeling.

Psychosomatic Illness:
Psyche means mental make-up, emotional profile. Soma means physical body. Psychosomatic illnesses express suffering on both levels. One cannot separate body from mind. Both are interconnected. If mind suffers, it would express in some physical illness. Physical disease can make mind fearful, depressed and anxious. It is difficult to decide whether an illness first starts in body and affects the mind later on, or whether it is the mental suffering that is reflected in the physical disease process. It would be safer to assume that any illness is the mixture of disturbance of the mind and the body, although the severity of mental and physical components could vary greatly. In psychosomatic illness, mind plays primary role in causation of physical disease. Disease affects whole person who has the mind as well as the body. Unless the mind and body are attended, the disease would not be controlled.

During my practice, I came across many cancer patients where I noticed unusual emotional distress. Later on, I realized that a majority of the patients had some emotional stresses. Cancer is not a psychological disease. However, many times there is undercurrent of mental distress due to unresolved conflicts. If doctors could search and try to help such issues, management of the disease becomes easier.

Giving adequate time to a patient and make him feel free to talk is the most important initial step. A sympathetic doctor, who can wisely spare adequate time to listen to the patient, wins half the battle even before actual treatment starts. Such doctors comprehend much more about the disease process than from mere recording of test findings, routine history and medical examination. "Look and thou shall find" is the famous saying from the Holy Bible. When a patient trusts the doctor, he will, knowingly or unknowingly, give a lot of helpful information about himself and about his disease.

Painful life events often trigger diseases, even a cancer process. Cancer is usually a disease of old age, by which time a man or woman has faced various stressful situations in life. Death of spouse, sudden death of a loved one, loss of job, retirement, financial ruins, rejection by own children or relatives, insults, worries about future of children are some practical problems, which create a lot of anxiety. Many people resolve the mental turmoil associated with such events. However, not everyone can cope up with such situation and such persons might express the mental suffering on a physical level in the form of a disease. Sometimes physical disease provides a subconscious escape route. Many life situations are practically hard to cope with while some others may be painful on subjective level. Many persons get delusions, illusions and distorted perceptions of situations, which may not have a realistic basis. The perceptions, however, are very real for the person who is experiencing such emotions and mental images.

It is my observation that homeopathic remedies work very well on many emotional problems and stressful situations. Homeopathy is a vast science. Chapters on "Mind" in homeopathy deal with various mental problems, which may be root causes of many illnesses. Homeopathy is a type of energy medicine. A homeopathic remedy may not have any actual material molecule to explain its' action on physical level but such a remedy carries an energy signature, a latent vibration, which might bring about the desired effect on the mental and physical levels. This chapter gives true stories of some of my cancer patients where we found significant interplay between mind and body. Treating the mind helped greatly in relief of symptoms. I do not suggest that homeopathy cures cancer. I know that homeopathic remedies can help greatly for symptomatic relief in certain psychosomatic situations. I will discuss my views on homeopathy for cancer in a later chapter.

This chapter gives some actual case histories. The names of the patients have been changed for the sake of confidentiality. All these patients were receiving conventional cancer therapy at Bombay Hospital in Mumbai. Homeopathic remedies were used only as a supplemental therapy after taking the consent from the patient or the relatives. During history taking, each patient was encouraged to come out with all his physical problems, emotional stress and painful life events if any. It was amazing to notice that given the sympathetic hearing and ample time, most of the patients could come out with significant incidents and peculiar feelings. After careful analysis of these symptoms by our homeopathic colleagues, appropriate remedies were quickly found with the help of a homeopathic software computer program. Selected remedies were given to the patients, who showed unusually rapid symptomatic improvement for each particular problem.

Case No. 1:
Vijaya, a 35 years old female patient developed headaches, vertigo, loss of appetite, drowsiness and stupor progressive over the previous 6 months. The patient was diagnosed to have Glioma of right thalamus, a brain tumor at the base of brain. The malignant nature of the tumor was confirmed by biopsy. The tumor, due to its' critical location could not be removed by operation. The patient was referred to me for radiation treatment, which was stared on Oct. 5th, 1993. She had persistent

headaches and the speech was disturbed. She did not show signs of improvement under radiation treatments.

Homeopathic assessment was done after two weeks. Patient was unmarried. She had an angry and haughty nature. She had developed headaches soon after her mother died in December 1992. In September1993, 9 months after her mother's death, she was diagnosed to have brain tumor seen on CT scan. Considering the totality of symptoms, Staphysagria-30 C was administered the homeopathic remedy. Within the next two weeks, there was more than 75% decrease in her headache, her speech improved markedly and her angry spells reduced markedly, as noticed by her relatives at home.

Case No. 2:
D.P. a 60-year-old male patient, who was a shopkeeper, was diagnosed to have prostate cancer in May 1991. This was treated with local radiation in an outside hospital in May/ June 1991. Patient responded well to this treatment and was free of pain till June 1993, when he suddenly developed severe pain in back and knees. He also complained of loss of weight, loss of appetite and he was depressed. The cancer had spread to bones as seen on bone scan. Hormone and chemotherapy did not help. Pain got worse in Oct. 1993, when he was referred to us at Bombay Hospital for radiation treatment for pain relief. His pain was not relieved in the first 2 weeks of radiation treatments.
During a personal conversation, when asked about his family, he almost broke down and said that his married daughter was murdered by a household servant in January 1993, after which he started getting backache and knee pains. Homeopathic assessment pointed to Ignatia 30 C, which was given mid-way during radiotherapy course. Within one week of getting Ignatia, patient showed more than 50% relief in pain and other symptoms.

Case No. 3:
This 69-year-old government officer had retired 10 years ago. He was doing part time consulting work. He slowly developed backache in 1991, which became worse and lead to severe sciatica type pain in Sept.

1993. Investigations at this time revealed a cancer tumor in lung, which has spread to bones in lower spine, pelvis and left hip. Unable to turn in bed, he was miserable with pain. He was referred to me for radiation treatment for pain relief.

Homeopathic history revealed that this man was active, cheerful and enjoyed his consulting work till sudden accidental death of his married son in a car accident in 1990. Patient's illness started after this incident. He was also anxious about his wife, who had some chronic health problems. Radiotherapy was started in Oct. 1993. Simultaneously, he was given Ignatia 30-C, a homeopathic remedy for grief reaction. There was dramatic return of cheerfulness within 4 days. His sadness decreased greatly. The backache, although still present, did not seem to bother him much.

Case No. 4:
Shabana, a 12 years old girl, had undergone partial removal of her brain tumor, parietal lobe astrocytoma, in August 1993. She was referred to me for post-operative radiotherapy, which was started on August 31st, 1993. She was depressed, fearful and complained of frequent headaches.

During a personal talk, Shabana disclosed that she was seeing a fierce looking black fakir following her on and off. She was greatly afraid of this man following her. She was getting scared and used to scream in sleep. This was a delusion well documented in homeopathic repertory. Stramonium 30-C s given to her on 13th Sept 1993, resulted in excellent improvement within one week. She became cheerful and headaches had gone. With a smile on her face, she told me in confidence that the black fakir had left chasing her.

Case No. 5:
Madhu, an eight-year-old little rowdy girl, developed sudden double vision, loss of balance and shaking of hands in August 1993. A CT scan revealed a tumor in the brain stem, which could not be operated because of its' critical location. Radiotherapy was started in Sept. 1993. This girl

was uncooperative, crying, screaming and restless. She used to throw temper tantrums.

Personal talk to her revealed that she lived outside Bombay and was brought to Bombay for medical treatment. She was homesick and irritable. She wept often when anything was refused to her. She told that she dreamt of ghosts often. Belladonna 30 was given as the chosen homeopathic remedy on 25th Sept 1993. On medical check up 2 weeks later, she was found to be cheerful and smiling. Her gait and coordination had improved greatly. She could now walk on her own without any support from others. She told that the ghost had almost stopped her visiting in dreams and anyway she was no longer scared of the ghosts!

Case number 1, 2 and 3 demonstrate unresolved grief reaction at the basis of physical suffering. Case number 4 and 5 reveal that delusions, fear of being persecuted and frightful visions play a significant role in the symptoms. There are many more cases on our record where such approach has worked well. Successfully addressing emotional turmoil goes a long way in the management of cancer. Homeopathy is able to play a significant complementary role in relieving underlying emotional disturbances.

Chapter 11

HOMEOPATHY FOR CANCER

Dr Samuel Hahnemann, a German physician, discovered the medical science of Homeopathy 200 years ago, in late 18th century. The World Health organization has recognized Homeopathy as a traditional system of medicine. W.H.O. has recommended its integration with conventional medicine for meeting the global needs for effective, safe and inexpensive health care by the year 2000!

Dr. Hahnemann experimented with himself and found that when he took daily doses of Cinchona Bark (a South American herbal medicine used for marsh fever), he developed symptoms like marsh fever. As soon as he stopped taking Cinchona, his symptoms subsided. He theorized that if large doses of a substance produced certain set of symptoms in healthy individuals, the same substance, in much diluted dose could cure the same symptoms in a diseased individual. He conducted such PROVINGS on himself and on many other healthy individuals. His experiments repeatedly confirmed his theory, which he called the Law of Similar. " Similia Similibis Curenter", which means Similar Cures Similar. Homeopathy means "Similar path or similar to disease pathology". Onions (allium cepa) cause watering and burning of eyes, therefore homeopathic allium cepa can cure eye inflammation, which presents with watering and burning as main symptoms. This concept is opposite of allopathy (allo= different, pathy=path), which in this case might use decongestants, antibiotics and steroids, medicines counteracting the symptoms. In a short span of few decades, hundreds of natural substances were thus proven and clinically tested. This led to the development of voluminous Homeopathic Materia Medica and Repertories, which form the basic references for the practice of Homeopathy.

Currently, an estimated 500 million people use homeopathic remedies annually worldwide for their health care. In Britain, homeopathic hospitals and clinics are part of their National Health System. Homeopathy is widely practiced all over Europe, especially in Germany and France. In India, there are about 25000 trained and licensed homeopathic practitioners helping millions of patients annually. Homeopathy was quite prevalent in USA in 19th century and early 20th century. With advent of pharmaceutical industry, homeopathy was thrown in the background. Philadelphia and Pittsburgh used to be important centers for development and practice of homeopathy till early 20th century. I was told that the Shady Side Hospital of Pittsburgh University was known as Hahnemann Homeopathic Hospital in the early part of this century.

How Does It Work?

There have been many controversies about how homeopathic remedies work. The homeopathic law states that " The more a remedy is diluted, the greater it's potency" This law apparently sounds ridiculous. In highly diluted form of a remedy above 12 - C potency, as per the Avagadro's Hypotheses, atoms of original substance cannot be detected. How can such a small or non-existent quantity of a substance produce any effects? Experiences of thousands of practitioners and millions of patients, however, vouch for the effectiveness and safety of homeopathy. If it were all due to PLACEBO EFFECT, as some of us would like to think, it would not work in infants or animals. Homeopathy is used effectively in infants and even in veterinary practice. This fact would put the question about placebo effect to the rest.

To understand how it may be working, we have to take support of quantum physics and theories developed by Albert Einstein. Mass and energy are interconvertible and there are many sub-atomic particles already known and many more remain to be discovered. Atom is no longer the smallest unit of matter. At sub-atomic level, a substance can and does leave its specific Vibratory Energy Signature in the carrier. This subtle vibratory energy can resonate with subatomic energy disturbances in the body, which may be the cause of the disease. It is therefore quite possible that these remedies are able to correct the subtle disease process and lead to effective cure of the physical disease process. Physics of Einstein has posed new challenges to old Newtonian theories, which stated that matter and energy are separate and cannot be inter-converted. As per Newtonian physics, atom was indivisible, a concept which has radically changed with advent of atomic physics in last century.

A recent study using nuclear magnetic resonance, M.R Scan Technology, demonstrated distinctive readings of sub-atomic activities in various highly diluted homeopathic remedies. These readings were absent in placebo. There are possibly specific electro-magnetic radiations emanating from homeopathic remedies, which may be counter-acting the subtle disturbances in the body. Some workers have theorized that homeopathic remedies create immune response and thus help the body cure itself. Anyway, as they say " the proof of pudding is in eating"!

Homeopathic treatment is directed towards the individual and NOT towards the any particular disease label. The same disease might require different remedies in different individuals, while one single remedy might also work for different diseases depending upon the constitution of the patients. According to homeopathy, " A disease is specific to the individual." This is holistic medical approach. Many times, if a proper remedy is chosen for a patient, it is seen that various layers of diseases, suffered by that person in the past, gradually unfold, come to surface and eventually get out of the system. Many a times, one single dose of a properly selected remedy can work wonders over a period of time. This way deeper disturbances are also taken care of effectively with homeopathy. This is known as Hering's Laws of Cure.

During my work at Jaslok Hospital in Bombay in 1970s, a surgical colleague Dr. B. P. Gandhi, FRCS, introduced me to homeopathy. While discussing some cases, Dr. Gandhi suggested names of some homeopathic remedies for pain control. The remedies were given to the patients, some of who showed dramatic pain relief over the next few days. We then tried some other remedies on more patients. I realized that homeopathic remedies are prescribed according to the constitution of a patient and not as per the disease. This medical science requires extensive study, deep understanding of the patient and peculiarity of his symptoms. I attended a special course in a local homeopathic medical college in Bombay to learn more about homeopathy.

In late 1980s and early 1990s, Dr. Lara Shah, a young homeopathic physician, helped us to conduct clinical trials on patients undergoing radiation treatments at Bombay Hospital. Dr. Shah used to assess a patient homeopathically and suggest some complementary homeopathic remedies. This combination apparently helped a large number of patients who seemed to be enthusiastic about this approach.

Homeopathy for Radiation Reactions:
We wanted to study if some of the homeopathic remedies were effective to reduce the radiation reactions and side effects. A patient under radiotherapy commonly develops loss of appetite, loss of energy, nausea, vomiting, abdominal cramps, diarrhea, pain while passing urine and stools. The reactions are variable and depend upon the part of the body under radiation treatment. We developed a protocol for a double blind clinical trial to compare the efficacy of two homeopathic remedies, Cobaltum and Causticum, against a placebo. In this trial, 82 patients undergoing radiotherapy were randomly divided in three groups. One group received placebo- dummy pills without any medicine. Second group was given causticum 30 and the third group cobaltum 30.

Causticum was selected because of its' actions on sadness, feeling of hopelessness, irritation, burning sensation, fatigue, rough sensations on mucous membranes and inflammation. Cobaltum was selected for its' actions on fatigue, pains, mood changes, abdominal pains, backache and mainly because of the fact that these patients were under cobalt radiation treatments.

Neither the doctors nor the individual patients knew which group a particular patient belonged. This was a double blind trial to do away with individual prejudices to prevent wrong conclusions. Each week, all the patients were checked up to see the progress and to record the level of radiation reactions. The trial went on for about 6 months. At the end, records were analyzed and conclusions drawn. These conclusions are given in following table. Compared to the placebo group whose reaction index was assigned as 100, cobaltum group had index of 55 and causticum group 63. This suggests a significant reduction in the severity of radiation reactions due to these two remedies in patients under radiation treatments.

Table Showing Severity of Radiation Reactions in the Three Groups: A, B and C.

Group	Remedy used	Number of Patients	Reaction Index	Reaction Level Reduction
A	Placebo	28	100	Baseline, N.A.
B	Cobaltum 30 C	26	55	45%
C	Causticum 30 C	28	63	37%

We did not observe any decrease in the effect off radiation treatment due to homeopathic supplements. In other words, homeopathic supplements neither interfered with action of radiotherapy nor enhanced radiation effect for better tumor regression. Following this trial, Cobaltum and Causticum were given to the patients routinely with their consent.

Homeopathy for Cancer:

Many papers and articles have been published about the possible use of homeopathy for cancer treatment. Various claims have been made. With my limited personal exposure to homeopathy, I cannot comment on the role of homeopathy in cure of cancer. However, I have observed homeopathy helping a great deal in many common acute and chronic medical diseases. In cancer, homeopathy can help for relief of symptoms although it may not directly act against the tumor process. Wrongly used, it can even stimulate tumor growth due to its' "Similar Cures Similar" philosophy. It is best to consult an experienced homeopathic physician before you consider any homeopathy for symptomatic relief or for long-term constitutional treatment to improve your immunity.

In the management of cancer, homeopathy can be used as a supportive treatment for give good relief from (1) Symptoms of cancer such as pain, restlessness, loss of sleep, fatigue, weakness, loss of appetite etc., (2) Symptoms of side reactions of cancer treatments such as nausea, vomiting, diarrhea, pain in abdomen, burning in urine, vertigo, weakness, etc and (3) for treatment of any other diseases unrelated to cancer or its' treatment.

Following is a list of some remedies we have found useful as a supplementary treatment. These are general observation. These can be used either in decimal 6X to 12X or centesimal 12 C to 200 C potency range. You should consult a homeopathic doctor before taking these remedies.

1. CONIUM: in 30 or 200 C potency can be given daily for 7 days initially with the beginning of radiation treatments. Keynotes: ailments in old age, hard tumors and glands, any swelling related to old injury, breast lumps and for cancer tendency.
2. PHOSPHORUS: in low potency 12 C or even 12X, can follow conium from second week of the treatment till the end of radiation course. Prevents weakness and exhaustion. Keynotes: burning spots, feeling of intense heat, great weakness and prostration, weariness, nausea, diarrhea, bleeding etc.

3. CAUSTICUM: Sometimes given in place of Phosphorus, when painful inflammation of mouth and throat is present with raw sensation due to radiation reaction.

4. IPECAC: Effective for nausea and vomiting related to radiotherapy and chemotherapy treatments. May be given 30 minutes prior to the treatment and repeated when required. Can be taken 30 minutes before meals to improve the appetite and reduce sensation of nausea to food.

5. PODOPHYLLUM: Given to control diarrhea resulting from radiation treatments to pelvis for lower abdominal cancers. If the diarrhea is not controlled, it might be advisable to give a gap of one or two weeks in the course of radiotherapy.

6. CANTHARIS: For severe burning in mouth, vagina, urethra and anal canal, cantharis liquid can be applied locally and also given orally. It is quite effective in temporarily relieving local burning pains.

7. CARCINOSIN: May be given as a single dose as a nosode before conventional treatment starts.

8. RADIUM BROMIDE 200-C: May be given to minimize the radiation reaction, daily for a few days.

There are many other homeopathic remedies, which can help under specific situations. You should undertake supplemental homeopathic treatments under a qualified homeopathic physician. WE have found that homeopathic remedies can be given simultaneously with other allopathic medicines without any adverse effects.

Classical homeopathy as developed by Samuel Hahnemann uses single remedies, which perfectly match the whole picture of the disease in a particular patient. The doctor observes patient's reaction over weeks and even months before a second prescription is given. This is a time consuming process but may produce good results at the hands of a good practitioner.

Combination Homeopathy:

Another current trend is to combine many different remedies in low potencies and administer the mixture to a patient on daily basis. Combinations produce quicker results in a variety of common conditions and may not require deeper case study of a patient. Many standard combinations for various common conditions are available in homeopathic medical stores. The components simultaneously work on a wide range of symptoms and organ systems. As far as I know, there is no specific combination for cancer, which is a difficult disease to treat. Many senior classical homeopathic doctors do not encourage combination homeopathy.

In Europe and USA, many homeopathic companies produce combination remedies for various purposes. Drainage remedies are low potency combinations that stimulate liver, intestines, kidneys, skin etc to improve their function. Detoxification remedies use medium potency combinations to dislodge the toxins from various tissues in body and bring these to be drained through the organs mentioned above. I have used some of these combinations during my work in USA and found these helpful to improve drainage, detoxification and immunity.

Although not a part of classical homeopathy, there are many other methods of using subtle extracts from various flowers, salts and plants. Bach flower remedies, Biochemic Remedies, Tissue Salts, Aromatherapy etc are some of these methods. A plethora of information is available on these methods in book form as well as on the Internet.

In conclusion, I can say that homeopathy is an effective, safe and gentle complementary method for improving quality of life of cancer patients. It can help a person for symptomatic relief. It should not be used as the only method to deal with cancer. Under guidance of a homeopathic physician, homeopathic remedies can be used simultaneously with other treatment methods.

Chapter 12

AYURVED FOR CANCER

Ayurved is the medical science developed in India more than 5000 years ago. Earliest available textbook, Sushrut Samhita, dates back to 700 B.C. Even in these early texts, references are given about still earlier texts, which are no longer available. As the tradition goes, Dhanwantari, The God of Medicine, is the originator of Ayurved, which is considered as the Fifth Veda. Ayurved is the science of health rather than science of disease. It stresses the preventive maintenance for good health, although it also suggests ways to overcome a disease. Ayurved is based on some fundamental concepts viz. Dosha, Agni, Dhatu, Mala and Ojas.

Hindu scriptures, *The Vedas,* state that the universe was created out of five elements called *pancha-maha-bho*ota. These elements are *Akash* (space), *Vayu* (air), *Tej* (fire), *Apa* (water) and *Prithvi* (earth). Before the creation, these elements were in a subtle invisible form. At the time of creation, first the Word (cosmic vibration) manifested. Other elements became sequentially manifest by process of *panchikaran* (inter-mixtures) of the invisible elements. The description about the creation of the universe is given in *Vedas* and other Hindu scriptures. Human body, which is miniature image of the universe, is also made out of the same five elements.

Dosha:

Combinations of panch-mahabhoota elements in a certain way produce what Ayurved calls as *Tridosha*, three constituents of the body. These three are *Vata, Pitta and Kapha*. When these three are in a proper balance, a person remains in good health. A disturbed dosha, when out of balance due to improper diet, habits and emotions, leads to ill health. The concept of dosha, although difficult to explain, is very important in understanding Ayurved. There is no synonym in English for dosha.

Kapha reflects qualities of earth and water and is responsible for stability of the body. It is the chief material constituent of the body. Kapha, whose constitution ranges from dense, unctous shleshak kapha to liquid state of tarpaka kapha, provides the basic building blocks for formation of new cells. It is the building material of the body. Kapha provides adhesive and cohesive forces to keep the body tissues together and in good condition. It is an anabolic factor. Technically, anabolic part of metabolism is responsible for building up the tissues, while the opposite catabolic part (catabolism) is responsible for cellular death and recycling of organic constituents. When Kapha is excessively disturbed, diseases like allergies, colds, coughs etc.

Pitta, which reflects the element Tejas- fire, is responsible for all the chemical activities of cells, heat in the body and bio-chemical activities. Pitta is responsible for intellect and for recycling of worn out cells. It is catabolic factor. Fever, heat, burning, ulcerations, infections are some of the manifestations of excessive pitta.

Vata, which reflects qualities of air and space, is responsible for all the movements and mobility of the body. Even movements of thoughts and emotions are controlled by vata. Vata also carries out all the commands for cell division and cell growth as well as for their recycling. Responsible for the functions of various organ systems, vata regulates the entire mind/ body apparatus. When Vata is disturbed, diseases affecting movements, such as arthritis, paralysis, loss of balance etc occur.

Above is a very simplistic explanation about only few common conditions arising out of dosha disturbances. In practice, dosha disturbance is a very complex subject leading to almost all the disease conditions. It is interesting to note that each of the dosha reflects the qualities of the parent elements from which it is made.

Agni:

Agni literally means fire and it represents Tejas Mahabhoota. In body, agni is responsible for digestion, assimilation and all the cellular biochemical activities. Agnis are thirteen in number, which work at three levels. Jatharagni is the primary- first level Agni, which digests food in stomach and intestines at a gross level. Good appetite expresses normal jathar- agni. Disturbed Agni could cause either too much or too poor appetite or appetite for wrong unhealthy foods. If food is not digested at this primary level due to disturbed Agni, a toxin termed Aama is formed. Undigested aama can disturb the doshas causing various diseases. Besides the main jatharagni, there are five mahabhootagni, each associated with each mahabhoota and seven dhatu-agni, one each with the seven dhatus. Mahabhootagni work at intermediate level and help convert food to more subtle nutrients for five sense organs associated with individual mahabhoota. Senses associated with panch mahabhoota respectively are: sound, touch, vision, taste and smell. Ears, skin, eyes, tongue and nose perceive these five senses, respectively. Finally, seven dhatu-agni help in metabolism of the nutrients at the cellular level.

Dhatu:
From the food we eat tissues are made. These tissues are named as *Dhatu* in Ayurved. Dhatu are seven in number and made up sequentially, each one from the preceding one. These seven dhatu are Rasa, Rakta, Mansa, Meda Asthi, Majja and Shukra. There are no exact anatomical equivalent terms for these seven dhatu. Grossly, rasa represents the digested fluid from which rakta (blood) is formed. Rasa also stands for lymph, a fluid circulating around all the cells. From blood, mansa (flesh) and from flesh meda (fat tissue) is formed. Further, from meda; asthi (bones), from asthi; majja (bone marrow) and from majja; shukra (fluid of vitality responsible for cellular rejuvenation and also for human reproduction) is formed. When all the dhatu are in pure healthy condition, body stays in good health. If disturbances in dosha persist over a long period of time, dhatu get contaminated with persistent dosha disturbances. Dhatu are also called as dooshya, since these are liable to get contaminated.

Mala:
Mala are waste products like stools, urine, sweat, menstrual discharge in women etc. Due to proper digestion and all the other processes

related to metabolism, proper quantities of mala are formed. These need to be discharged from the body. This is a detoxification process.

Ojus:
Ojus is the subtle principle that reflects vitality, intelligence and strength. Ojus cannot be shown in any material form, although it expresses in all the life activities.

Ayurvedic Concept of Cancer:
According to ayurved, there is no specific single disease termed as cancer. Cancer is a group of chronic disorders related to long term uncorrected disturbance affecting various dhatu and dosha. Cancer could manifest as a predominantly local disease in the form of an arbuda or granthi, the Sanskrit terms for tumor. Cancer can manifest even as a non-healing ulcer, dushta vrana. Cancer could have additional symptoms of a systemic disease such as loss of weight, weakness, chronic fever and other disturbances. Ayurvedic diagnosis of cancer may differ in different patients diagnosed to have same histological type of cancer confirmed by modern medical techniques. Assessment of dosha, dhatu and Agni are important for establishing ayurvedic diagnosis. Ayurved recommends the treatment according to the patient's constitution and as per the specific disturbances in dosha and dhatu found on ayurvedic assessment of the patient.

Ayurvedic Diagnosis:
Ayurvedic methods of diagnosis are 1. Trividha Pariksha: Inspection, Palpation and Questioning about the disease history. 2. Ashtavidha (eight fold examination) of which examination of tongue and nadi (pulse) is important. 3. Indriya Pariksha: examination of individual organs, 4. Srotasa Pariksha: Examination of various systems and channels, and finally 5. Nidan Panchak: five fold final deliberations to decide the exact cause, progress, prognosis and treatment of disease.

In earlier times, modern tests like blood test, X-rays, scan etc were not known. However, modern day Ayurvredic physician takes all the help from these tests for diagnosis and treatment of a patient.

Ayurvedic Treatment:
For disease prevention, Ayurved outlines appropriate Ahara (foods), Vihara (life style) and Vichara (thought process). These recommendations vary from person to person and from season to season. Detailed recommendations are given in ayurvedic texts on this subject. The emphasis is on prevention of the disease. However, if a disease starts, ayurvedic treatment is based on following methods:

These treatment methods are:

1. SHODHAN, Panch Karma: Detoxification and purifications of various tissues and organs. Panch-Karma are five-fold methods employed for Shodhan. These are preceded by Poorva-Karma Snehan and Swedan (i.e. medicated oil massage and steam baths). One or more of the 5 Pancha-Karmas then follow in a daily session, which goes on for 1 or 2 weeks.

2. SHAMAN: Pacification and re-balancing of your defective dosha, usually with some herbal and mineral remedies.

3. RASAAYAN: Rejuvenation of body tissues for maintenance of youth and increasing immunity.

Ayurvedic medicines are prepared from natural substances like herbs, minerals, metals and animal products. There are elaborate guidelines to prepare various products, which are usually made from multiple constituents.

Modern medical scientists often wonder about the " Active Principle" in ayurvedic products. We cannot apply the same yardsticks to ayurvedic products as applied to modern pharmaceutical products, which are mostly manufactured as synthetic molecules in a laboratory. Each herb might have a variety of active molecules working synergistically on various levels. We have to believe in Nature's intelligence in producing a medicinal herb, which might have many "active principles" mutually enhancing beneficial effects while keeping away toxic effects of individual alkaloids, polypeptides, polysaccharides or whatever name pharmaceutical industry discovers for such " Active Principles"! It is neither possible nor advisable to subject each herb to a series of chemical analytical tests, which would decrease the holistic effect of any natural product. Besides being ecologically dangerous, such practices would skyrocket the cost of herbal medicines making them unaffordable to a common man. Most of these herbal products, being used over many centuries, have been found to be safe and effective. The benefits of such herbal products could always be reconfirmed by well-designed limited clinical trials on actual patients. Unlike modern pharmaceuticals, these natural products have a wide safety margin. The real test of the pudding is in eating. New medicines based on personal experiences of leading Ayurvedic consultants are also being added from time to time.

Ayurvedic Research at Wagholi:

Since early 1980s, I was studying complementary medicine with a view to reduce radiation reactions and to improve quality of life of my patients. My mother Dr. Laxmibai Kulkarni was a well-known ayurvedic practitioner in Pune in 1930s and 40s. Securing a gold medal, she ranked first in her final examination for the Ayurvedic medical degree. In my childhood, I naturally got exposed to various herbs and ayurvedic preparations. Sometimes I used to accompany her when she visited patients. My father, Mr. Nanasaheb Kulkarni, had a shop in Pune to sell medicinal herbs and chemicals. Since my early childhood, I had decided to become a doctor. During my allopathic medical training, I almost forgot about ayurved. Later on after many years into my practice as radiation oncologist in Mumbai, Vaidya Bhave rekindled my latent interest as mentioned in the preface of this book.

In early 1980s, I came into contact with Sardeshmukh Maharaj and his family. Maharaj was a saintly figure, whose mission was to promote ancient Indian sciences and arts. It was very inspiring and interesting to spend time with Maharaj, who was always eager to instruct us about Ayurved. Previous seven generations in Sardeshmukh family were well known for practicing Ayurved in Maharashtra. Sardeshmukh Maharaj, who himself excelled in Nadi-Pariksha (Ayurvedic pulse analysis), passed on this rare skill to his children, especially to the oldest son Dr. Sadanand Sardeshmukh. Maharaj established the Bharatiya Sanskriti Darshan Trust in early 1960s to promote the Indian Sciences and Arts. A spacious 60 acres of land was acquired at Wagholi, 15 miles east of Pune in foothills of Maharashtra, for the work of this institution.

I often met with Maharaj and Dr. Sardeshmukh to discuss about utility of ayurved in cancer. I referred some of my cancer patients to Dr. Sardeshmukh for complementary ayurvedic treatment, which seem to help a significantly for symptomatic relief and improving general condition. In 1986, Maharaj directed us to develop a Cancer Project with Ayurvedic line of treatment. Further trials on individual patients were conducted over the next few years. Finally in April 1994, the Cancer Research Project was launched at Ayurvredic Hospital and Research Center at Wagholi and soon extended to Mumbai and Solapur with help of Dr Shirish Kumthekar, a cancer surgeon.

Sardeshmukh Maharaj left this world in 1996. His vision is now unfolding and the mission expanding. With ceaseless efforts of Sardeshmukh family and help from dedicated staff and friends, various projects are blooming as envisaged by Sardeshmukh Maharaj. Besides the Ayurvedic Hospital and Research Center, magnificent Panch-karma Cottages, an Ayurvedic Medical College and an Ayurvredic Pharmacy are providing many unique services in this holy location. Standing at distance, Maharaj Sardeshmukh's Samadhi Shrine provides constant blessings and inspiration to the visitors. Recently, a beautiful Matha (monastery) building has been added to promote Spiritual Practices, Yoga and Indian Classical Music.

The Cancer Research Project:

Started in 1994, this project has enrolled about 1200 cancer patients between 1994 and 2001. Cancer patients with biopsy confirmed diagnosis of cancer are accepted to join this project. Patients are initially given the detailed idea about the project with possible scope and possible limitations of Ayurvedic treatment for cancer. A patient is required to sign written consent showing his acceptance to join the project. A patient can withdraw from the project anytime for any reason. A dedicated team of ayurvedic and allopathic doctors working in this project record detailed history and all the reports of the patient. Patient with any type of cancer is accepted in the project as long as he can attend regular follow-ups. History and progress reports are recorded in ayurvedic as well as allopathic format. Patients are then divided in four groups as follows:

Group A: Freshly diagnosed cancer patients who wish to try only Ayurvedic treatment initially.
Group B: Patients who have already tried major surgery, radiotherapy, chemotherapy as first treatment of the cancer, but treatment failed.
Group C: The patients, currently undergoing chemotherapy and / or radiotherapy, who wish to take complementary ayurvedic treatment.
Group D: The patients, whose cancers have been controlled due to allopathic treatment for more than 6 months, wishing to take complementary ayurvedic treatment in addition.

Initially, a detailed medical examination is performed on each patient to decide the extent of cancer. Ayurvedic pulse diagnosis, nadi pariksha forms an important part of the examination. Ayurvedic line of treatment is decided for each patient, who is reviewed once a month or more frequently if needed. Patients who need panch-karma treatments are instructed accordingly. All the patients receive oral medicines for daily consumption. The medicines are periodically changed as per the progress of the case. Every year, all the case records are subjected to statistical analysis, after which yearly reports are published about the observations and results. Common ayurvedic medicines used in this project are as follows:

Churna: (Herbal powders, either single or mixtures): Ashwagandha, Shatavari, Gokshura, Ananta, Vasa, Yashtimadhu, Kankole, Haridra, Lodhra, Arjuna, Pushkarmul, Raktarohitaka, Sharapunkha, Triphala, Sitopaladi, Talisadi, Hingvashtak churna.

Vati/ Guti- (Tablets): Arogyavardhini, Chandraprabha, Laxmivilas, Shankhavati, Pravalpishti, Praval Panchamrut, Kamadudha, Asthiposhak, Triphalvati

Avaleha (Syrup): Vasavaleha, Dadimavaleha, Bilvavaleha.

Guggul Kalpa (Tablets): Guggul, Lakshadi guggul, Gokshuradi guggul, Kanchanar guggul, Triphala guggul, and Mahayogaraj guggul.

Asava-Arishta (Liquids, Decoctions): Kumari asav, Varunadi kwath,

Siddha Ghrut: (Medicated ghee-clarified butter): Yashtimadhu ghrut, Dadimadi ghrut, Padmakadi ghrut

Siddha Taila- (Medicated oils): Anu taila, Yashtimadhu taila, Irimedadi taila, Nimba taila, Durvadi taila, Chandan-bala-lakshadi taila, Karanja taila, Bahubija taila,

Kalpa (Powders): Shatavari kalpa, Badam pak, Anant kalpa

Suvarna Kalpa (Tablets/Powders): Raupya suvarna sootashekhar, Suvarna sootashekhar, Suvarna malini vasant, Brihat vata chintamani

Patient is instructed about specific diet regimes (Pathya) to avoid dosha-disturbing foods in each particular case. No guarantee is given for any cure. Mental stress, an important factor in cancer, is assessed and ways to reduce this stress are discussed. In acute cases, follow up is done at weekly interval. Thereafter, patients are called once a month. X-rays, blood tests and scans are repeated frequently to confirm the progress of the case. This treatment is continued for about three years. Thereafter, maintenance treatment with Rasayana (rejuvenation) anti-ageing medicines is prescribed on long-term basis as per the needs of each case.

Observations:

Ayurvedic line of supportive treatment is highly beneficial for improving general condition, for pain relief and for reducing side reactions of chemotherapy and radiotherapy. More than 80% of the patients in this trial had very advanced stage cancer, which were not controlled by prior allopathic treatments. Ayurvedic treatment, although not found curative on its' own, was helpful to give good symptomatic relief in a great majority of cases. Chemotherapy / radiotherapy reactions in patients of C group were reduced by 40% to 60%. Conventional treatments as surgery, radiotherapy and chemotherapy should be used as the primary treatment for removing or reducing cancer tumor and Ayurvedic treatment should be used as a supplement to improve quality of life and to give better symptomatic relief.

For more information of this center at Wagholi, please log on www.ayurved-wagholi.org

Conclusion:

I have described one of the cancer projects with which I am associated. We have found that Ayurved is a very important line of complementary treatment for cancer. This natural science analyses the individual's prakriti (constitution) and dosha disturbances, which are at the root of any disease process. Ayurved emphasizes on disease prevention through restoration of healthy life styles and food habits. It balances the internal environments in the body enabling it to resist disease process. It has important methods for body purification, detoxification, restoration of disturbed dosha and for cellular rejuvenation. Using mostly natural time tested products, ayurvedic treatments are safe, effective and affordable. Ayurvedic treatments are directed not so much against the cancer tumor but for strengthening the immune system.

There are many more ayurvedic practitioners and ayurvedic research centers actively involved in cancer research. The views from various centers would certainly add more to the understanding of ayurvedic treatment in cancer. You should consult an experienced ayurvedic practitioner before undertaking any supplementary ayurvredic treatment for your cancer problem.

Chapter 13

UNUSUAL CANCER PATIENTS

In this chapter, I propose to illustrate some true stories of cancer patients. There are many patients who have shown unusual courage to fight cancer. There are some others who showed rapid development of cancer with unexpected deterioration. The same treatment given for same stage of cancer in different patients may not produce same results, which are variable due to undisclosed or unknown factors. Many patients, worried about adverse comments from orthodox medical practitioners, did not initially tell what extra efforts they were taking to deal with the disease. A cancer patient wants to get cured as soon as possible by whatever means he believes would help. The relatives are ready to go to any extent to try new methods and new medicines, which might not have been proved to help in cancer. In such a hurry, sometimes there can be a danger of submitting to a worthless treatment or even a harmful treatment. Everyday, some well-wishers suggest some new miracle medicine. With the advent of Internet surfing, one could get easily submerged in a sea of information on the web. It is hard and confusing to sort out what could be useful in an individual situation. It is best to have some sympathetic and experienced doctor to consult in such matters for the right advice. Many things may be working but one individual cannot undertake too many methods at one time.

Following true stories, which defy the statistics, could be interesting since each one illustrates certain subtle points. The names of the patients have been changed for the sake of professional confidentiality. Most are the stories of my own patients, although some stories are quoted from other doctors and their published works.

1. A throat cancer survivor:

Vishwanath, a retired professor, developed cancer of throat (supraglottic area) in 1975 when he was 65 years old. He was examined in a cancer hospital in Mumbai and was advised to take a full course of radiation treatments. Since the patient was from Pune, he took the treatments in Pune. He developed moderate radiation reactions, which subsided after 4 weeks from the end of radiotherapy. He was re-examined and was told that his cancer has disappeared. After about 1 year, Vishwanath noticed a gland in the left side of the neck, which was due to spread of the cancer to the lymph node. At this time, he consulted me at the Bombay Hospital. I examined and found that the cancer had recurred in the throat and had spread to the lymph nodes in the neck. The patient, who thought he was cured, was disappointed. At this time a second course of radiotherapy was given to the neck area. The patient, who was very cooperative and a noble person, faithfully completed the second course of radiation, which was planned carefully to avoid overexposure of radiation. At the end of radiation, the nodes shrunk more than 75% and the throat tumor more than 60%.

He was anxious about the future health. At this time, Dr. B.G Wad had done research on Bhallatak (semicarpus anacardium) in Mumbai. An oral jelly from this herbal nut, Anacarcin, was marketed by Bombay Pharmaceutical Company. I suggested the patient to take this medicine twice daily for 6 months. Fortunately, at the end of 6 months I found that the neck node and the throat tumor both had almost disappeared. Encouraged by the results, I advised the patient to continue Anacarcin for some more time. Vishwanath eagerly continued Anacarcin for the next 5 years. On regular check ups till 1980, he was found to be in very good health, good spirits and free of any nodes or cancer tumor. He passed away at the age of 80 years due to a sudden heart attack, unrelated to his cancer.

It is not unusual to control an early stage throat cancer with radiotherapy alone. However in this case, cancer had come back and spread to the nodes within first year after radiotherapy. Under this situation, chances of cure were very minimal. I believe that Anacarcin and the patient's faith in the treatment were mainly responsible for the cure.

2. A boy with fibro-sarcoma- a cancerous tumor under the skin:

Pramod, a 12-year-old boy was brought to me by his father at Jaslok Hospital in 1973. This boy had twice undergone operations to remove a tumor on the left arm in the previous year. Unfortunately, the tumor had recurred at the same place within 8 months after the operation. It was again operated but was likely to recur if nothing else was done. After examination, I advised a course of local radiation to the operated area to minimize chance of relapse. Patient completed the course of radiation within the next few weeks. At that time, we were trying some ayurvedic medicine orally and ayurvedic oil for local application. Patient continued on this supplementary treatment for more than a year. At regular follow-ups over the next five years, he was found to be in good health and free of cancer. We still meet occasionally as good friends. This boy, who had philosophical inclinations from the childhood, has now become a Sanyasin and pursues a religious life helping other devotees in an ashram in Pune. It is now more than 30 years since his initial diagnosis of tumor.

I feel that in addition to radiotherapy, supplementary ayurvedic treatment, faith and religious orientation prompting this boy on the path of meditation and yoga has helped tremendously to overcome the disease.

3. Meenaben, a woman who had cancer of left ear:

Meenaben, a 60 years old pleasant and righteous woman from Gujarat, was operated at Bombay Hospital in 1992 for a cancer in the left ear. The ear and the surrounding bone were removed and she no longer could hear on the left side. She was referred to me for a post-operative course of radiotherapy that was completed in Feb. 1992. The patient was very careful about her health and came for yearly follow-ups for the next 10 years all the way from her native place. In the last follow up in Feb. 2002, I was happy to see her in good spirits and good health and no evidence of recurrence of cancer. In between she did have some transient complaints like cataract, arthritis, urinary infections etc that were cured.

Recently, learning about my interest in holistic medicine, she triumphantly mentioned the secret of her good health. She was taking water therapy that she thought helped her to bring down her high blood pressure. She also mentioned about an ayurvedic herb from Gujarat, Krishnavalli, which she had been taking since her treatment in 1992. She even sent me an old Gujarathi transcript, which she found in her old family treasures, about the properties of this herb. She wanted me to experiment with this herb for cancer treatment. When we got to know each other better, I learnt that she was a regular practitioner of Yoga, Pranayama and Meditation. I am sure all these complementary methods have gone a long way in controlling her cancer over the past 10 years.

4. Shobha with cancer of uterus:

I met this active woman in 1977, when she was only 32 years old. She had advanced cancer of uterus for which we gave her a short course of radiation at Bombay Hospital before the operation by Dr. B. N. Purandare to remove her uterus. Soon after the operation, remaining half of radiation treatment was also administered. We advised supplemental ayurvedic treatment to minimize her radiation reactions and to improve her general condition. She comes regularly for check-ups, the last one being in December 2001, almost 24 years since her initial diagnosis of cancer. She has been disease free and in very good health all threes years. I again feel that her positive attitude, faith and ayurvedic supplemental medicines have helped her a great deal in the cure of her disease.

5. Bansidhar, a case of cancer of esophagus, `(food-pipe):

This 45 years old businessman from Secundarabad received radiation treatment at Bombay Hospital in 1980 for his advanced cancer of the middle part of esophagus. A jovial and energetic man, Bansidhar had positive attitude to look at all the things in the life. I instructed him to prepare Bhallatak (Semicarpus anacardium) medicinal milk at his home for daily consumption. He followed the instructions carefully and cheerfully. He used to come for regular check ups over the next 10 years and we found that his cancer had completely disappeared as confirmed by repeated x-ray tests. He had no problem for eating and was doing his business as usual. Cancer of esophagus is a dangerous disease, not easy to control. I believe bhallatak milk has helped him greatly in addition to his cheerful attitude.

6. Vinayak, another case of cancer of esophagus, (food-pipe):

This 60 years old man started a course of 9 cycles of chemotherapy in Mumbai in Jan 1998, for his cancer of food-pipe. He joined our Ayurvedic Cancer Project and started attending Dr. Sardeshmukh's clinic in Mumbai right from the beginning of the chemotherapy. Vinayak's mother, brother and sisters had various cancers indicating strong family history of risk for cancer. Because of this background, he was anxious to do all he could to cure his cancer. With simultaneous supplemental ayurvedic treatments, he tolerated the strong chemotherapy sessions fairly well without any severe side effects. After the completion of chemotherapy course, he was given radiotherapy course at some other hospital in Mumbai. Over the past 3 years, he does not have any cancer seen on his x-rays and scans. At the last check up in May 2002, he was found to be in good health and busy in his usual activities. He is now kept on Rasayana ayurvedic medicines as a preventive measure.

7. A cancer patient who responded to water injections:

From the book " Love, Medicine and Miracles" by Bernie Siegel, M.D., I quote the following dramatic story about the role of positive attitude and faith in the treatment of cancer. Mr. Wright, a patient in New York suffering from advanced cancer of lymph nodes (lympho-sarcoma), was under the treatment of Dr. Klopfer in 1957. Mr. Wright had developed orange sized multiple nodes in neck, armpits, groins, chest and abdomen. All the known treatments had proved ineffective. The liver and the spleen were enormously enlarged. His lungs used to pour milky water in chest that had to be removed frequently with aspiration. He had to have oxygen to breath and he was on heavy doses of sedations. Despite his bad condition, Mr. Wright had great hope.

At that time a new drug, Krebiozen, was being tested for cancer treatment. It was an experimental drug and Mr. Wright did not qualify to receive this trial drug because of his terminal cancer condition. However, at the insistence of the patient, Dr. Klopfer was successful in obtaining this drug for Mr. Wright. A wonder happened when this trial medicine was given to Mr. Wright, who soon started to walk around the ward, chatting happily with the nurses. Mr. Wright's nodes started melting like butter and within 10 days his tumors vanished, his condition became normal and he was discharged from the hospital. He took off in his own aeroplane and flew at height of 12000 feet quite comfortably.

Mr. Wright was all right for a few months when doubts about Krebiozen started appearing in the newspapers, which greatly disturbed him. Mr. Wright soon developed recurrence of his lymphosarcoma. His condition rapidly worsened. Dr. Klopfer, curious to investigate this further, told the patient that some shipments of the trial drug were defective hence there were some doubts. The doctor further told the patient that a new shipment of the drug would soon arrive. Mr. Wright was greatly relieved by this reassurance. He was ecstatic to learn that the new injections would be started on him in a couple of day's time. With much fanfare, the pure version of the drug, (in reality distilled water), was given as injections. The results were dramatic with even better shrinkage of the nodes and marked improvement in health from his "terminal state"! Water injections were continued since these worked wonders. He was all right for the next two months when finally the American Medical Association published a report that Krebiozen was really worthless in cancer treatment. This proved to be a heart breaking news for Mr. Wright, who suddenly started deteriorating. His cancer nodes came back and he passed away within the next few days.

There are many more intriguing true stories about cancer. I am sure most of the doctors, who have treated cancer patients, would be able to narrate unusual stories about their patients. The simple truth is, happy people generally don't get sick. One's attitude towards oneself is the single most important factor in staying healthy and preventing disease. Faith plays a great role.

Reviewing a large number of cancer patients who were " spontaneously cured", Canadian Professor Dr. Harold Foster found in 1988 that most of these patients had made major dietary changes– usually switching to vegetarian diet and avoiding white flour, refined sugars and canned foods, before the "cure" happened!
I believe that positive optimistic attitude coupled with complementary treatments combined with judicious use of conventional methods would go a long way in reversing cancer process and produce much better results. If you wish to read more stories about unusual cancer patients, please refer to following books:

1. Love, Medicine & Miracles, by Bernie Siegel, M.D., (Arrow Publication)
2. A Definitive Guide to Cancer, Alternative Therapies, by Burton Goldberg, W. John Diamond & W. Lee Cowden; (Future Medicine Publishing, Inc)
3. Manifesto For A New Medicine, by James S. Gordon, M.D., (Perseus Books)
4. Options, The Alternative Cancer Therapy Book, by Richard Walters, (Avery Publishing)

Chapter 14

Frequently Asked Questions

Q. 1. Can you cure cancer?

A: If you ask me whether I can cure YOUR cancer, the answer is NO. The cure of any disease has to come from within the patient. Doctors and medicines only help the patient to fight his own battle. Hence, the modified answer to your question is: "Yes, together we two can reverse the process of cancer hopefully leading to a cure." One should however remember that cancer is a complex disease process caused by a variety of factors as explained in earlier chapters of this book. Sometimes, patients have negative attitude, hopelessness and mental blocks in the process of healing. In cancer, modern medicine states 5-year survival rate, rather than call it a cure. This generally means that if a cancer is controlled for 5 years, the chances of it coming back are very remote (although not impossible). Further a cancer patient could develop other diseases also, which could take the toll. Death is the other side of the coin we call life. We should make all the efforts to accept the challenge of cancer and do everything to improve the quality of life.

Q. 2. Doctors told me that my 2 years old son probably has leukemia. It has come as a shock to the whole family. What can we do now?

A: This is a very tragic situation, especially for the parents and family members. Doctors will conduct some more tests to determine the type of leukemia and its stage. Leukemia is a disease of white blood cells. The usual treatment for childhood leukemia is intensive chemotherapy for a few months followed by low dose chemotherapy for a couple more years. Some children are given radiation treatments to brain to minimize chances of leukemia spreading to brain. All these treatments are very toxic and produce a lot of side effects. In more than 80% patients, such treatments produce what we call a remission, which means no evidence of leukemic cells in the blood or body. You have to consider taking complementary treatment to support the general condition of the child during these trying times. If you refuse to undergo chemotherapy treatment for whatever reasons, you should consider complementary treatments with Ayurved, Herbs, and Nutrition etc. Complementary treatments do not guarantee any definite cure but these could be safer and less toxic to the patient. Some Ayurvedic practitioners claim good results in leukemia but the mainline oncologists might not agree with this view. Finally, you have to decide for yourself what treatment options you wish to try.

Q. 3. My father has got a cancer of food-pipe diagnosed recently. He is 70 years old and he does not wish to take any treatment. We are forcing him to get admitted to a cancer hospital for operation. Please advise how we can handle this situation.

A: Cancer of esophagus (food-pipe) is usually diagnosed at late stage since the symptoms are vague and not attended to promptly. If the cancer is in early stage, which has not spread to lymph nodes or distant organs, major operation to remove the cancer has a fair chance of controlling the disease. Many times, during the operation, the surgeon finds that the cancer is too advanced and cannot be removed. Careful examination and medical tests should guide the surgeon to decide about the operation. Even after a successful operation, a course of chemotherapy and/ or radiotherapy would be usually recommended. Five-year survival rates for this type of cancer after conventional treatments are reported to be less than 10%. Please feel free to discuss with your doctors about chances of cure, side effects, expenses etc. beforehand. You should consider all these factors before making up your mind. However, the choice to either accept the operative treatment or decline it is entirely with the patient and his family. Your father is 70 years old and must have gone through a lot of experiences in his life. I can understand your anxiety to see your father get all the treatments recommended by your doctors. I suggest you do not force your father in making a decision he does not like in his heart. Let him decide what he wishes to do, after considering all the pros and cons of various options. I am not aware of your economic conditions to withstand all these expensive treatments. That should also be a factor in your decision-making.

Q. 4. My 56 years old brother developed pain in abdomen 2 months ago. A CT scan was recently taken and the doctors say it could be cancer of pancreas. Will operation cure this cancer?

A: Cancer of pancreas is a dangerous disease and usually inoperable. If the tests show that it can be completely removed by operation, this would help. Discuss all your questions about chances of cure, other treatments, expenses etc with your surgeon. You need also to take nutritional and other complementary therapies to support the patient during his illness. These are discussed at length in earlier chapters.

Q. 5. What is your opinion about Auto-urine therapy? Does it work?

A: Auto-urine therapy means drinking your own urine for treatment of your illness. The idea of auto-urine therapy could be repulsive for majority of the patients. I personally would not recommend it to my patients. However, if a patient is keen to try this, I have no objection. I have seen many patients who undertake such treatments and have subjectively reported good benefits. When a patient is on many medications, their breakdown products are excreted in urine. I do not know whether drinking such urine would be harmful or helpful. There are many books written on this subject in local languages as well as in English, which might give you more information. Mentioned in ancient Indian medical books as Shivambu Chikitsa, urine therapy was advocated by many prominent persons, including the former Prime Minister of India, Mr. Morarji Desai. Recently, Dr. Burzinski from Texas has discovered some polypeptides in human urine, which he termed as antineoplaston. Antineoplastons apparently help to shrink some cancer tumors. Other workers are giving urea, a substance found in urine, to treat liver cancer. This is a controversial topic. I would not be able to say whether or not urine therapy works in cancer treatment.

Q. 6. My mother is under cycles of chemotherapy for breast cancer. She is getting a lot of nausea and vomiting. Her skin and nails have got black spots. She gets burning sensation in body and feet. She is worried about loss of hair. Should she continue chemotherapy?

A: Without knowing all the details of the patients, especially stage and type of cancer, her general condition and response to earlier treatments, it would be difficult for me to give you any definite answers. Is this a palliative chemotherapy for her recurrent cancer or is it a routine post-operative preventive chemotherapy? Has the cancer been earlier operated successfully? What is her general condition like? Are her reactions very severe or mild? Does she wish to continue chemotherapy? When there is persistent cancer spread in the body, chemotherapy usually does not help much. Chemotherapy might be able to produce some temporary shrinkage of tumor, which is likely to come back. You need to discuss all these issues with your doctors and then take a wise decision. Regardless of what decision you might take, I would suggest the patient should have supportive nutritional, herbal and ayurvedic treatments to reduce the side reactions and to improve the quality of life.

Q. 7. I am working as a teacher. My wife suffers from cancer of stomach for past 3 months. She was operated but they could not remove the cancer tumor. They have now advised chemotherapy and told me that I should be prepared to spend about Rs 10000 per month for the next 6 months. It is very hard for me to gather that kind of money. Further the doctors say that there is no guarantee of any cure. I am scared. Please advice.

A: I am sorry to hear about the difficult situation you are facing. There is no effective chemotherapy for stomach cancer. At most, chemotherapy might produce temporary shrinkage of the tumor. You say that the stomach cancer could not be completely removed at the operation. Considering the nature of the disease, toxic effects of chemotherapy with no hope for cure and your economic hardship, it would be all right if you declined the chemotherapy. You should discuss this matter with your wife and give due consideration to her wishes. Please discuss all this aspects with the doctor who has recommended the chemotherapy treatments. Even if you decline chemotherapy, you should keep trying some of the complementary medical options, which might afford comparable or even better results. Please trust God and have faith. Miracles can happen. With positive attitude and all the support from the family, your wife can reverse the process of cancer.

Q. 8. Can you suggest any treatment for reducing reactions to chemotherapy?

A: Chemotherapy reactions are a common problem, dreaded by the patients. However, not everyone under chemotherapy gets severe reactions. Many patients tolerate chemotherapy complaining only mild side reactions. It depends mostly on the drugs and dosages used for chemotherapy and upon the constitution of the patient. Seen from Ayurvedic point of view, Pitta Prakriti (constitution) patients get more severe reactions than Kapha types. Lot of fluids and nutritional supplements with vitamins A, B-Complex, C, D and E would help reduce the degree of reactions. Praval-pishti, an organic calcium preparation from sea coral has a cooling effect, which reduces the intensity of reactions. Praval-pishti, two tablets twice daily can be taken during the course of chemotherapy. There are many more effective Ayurvedic medicines to help reduce reactions, for which you need to consult an Ayurvedic practitioner. Complaints like nausea, vomiting, pain etc can also be effectively controlled by some allopathic medications, which your doctors would prescribe.

Q. 10: Is there any certain treatment in Ayurved for cancer?

A: As far as I am aware, there is no certain treatment in ayurved to cure cancer. Cancer is a complex disease resulting from long-term constitutional and genetic disturbances. Ayurved tries to restore the normal functioning of organs and enable body to fight disease. It does not have any specific medicines to kill the cancer cells directly. Ayurved has a definite role to play as a supplemental therapy in overall management of cancer disease. Some traditional Ayurvedic practitioners report good results with Heerak Bhasma (made from diamond). There are many other claims associated with other formulae.

Q.11. The doctor giving radiation treatment to my father got angry with us since we were giving some Ayurvedic medicines side by side without the doctor's knowledge. He says this has spoilt the case. My father is now worried. What can we do to please the doctor?

A: It would have been good if you had informed the doctor about the Ayurvedic medicines you are giving your father during radiation treatment. Open-minded doctors would try to get more information about other systems rather than get angry with the patients in such situations. In our experience, Ayurvedic medicines do not "spoil" the cases, rather if used properly, "help" the cases. Try to discuss this matter with the doctor without being worried. Do not be intimidated. After all, it is the health of your father, which is at stake. As a last resort, you may even look for a better doctor, who is open-minded and more sympathetic.

Q. 12. Should we take large doses of vitamin C and Vitamin E during chemotherapy cycles, as suggested by a friend who herself underwent chemotherapy cycles a few months ago?

A: As per the recent research, large doses of vitamin C (1000 to 2000 mg daily) and natural vitamin E (200 to 400 mg daily) during chemotherapy are found to be beneficial. These vitamins are effective in 1. Counteracting damaging free radicals that are liberated during chemotherapy. 2. Help maintain normal tissue function and oxygenation of cells. 3. Possibly enhance effects of chemotherapy. Linus Pauling, the Nobel Laureate, advocates very high doses of vitamin C to help cure many diseases. Vitamin C is given in very large doses (10000 to 15000 mg) through intravenous drips in some Alternative Medical Centers abroad. This has to be done under strict medical supervision. For an average patient, oral consumption of vitamins in doses given in the beginning should suffice.

Q. 13. We want to give best treatment to our father who has been diagnosed to have lung cancer. My sister lives in America. We want to know if taking him to America will help?

A: I am happy to note that you wish to do everything possible for your father. There are various points to consider for an Indian wishing to take treatment in USA. India is fortunate to have very well trained doctors and excellent hospitals with all the medical facilities. In fact, Indian doctors are highly regarded in USA, UK and other countries for their knowledge, intelligence and hard work. All the major cities in India offer excellent medical facilities and well-trained doctors, which are comparable to hospitals abroad.

The medical treatment in USA is very expensive. Without health insurance, even local Americans cannot afford to go to hospitals. What is your economic situation? Has your sister asked your father to come to America for treatment or is this your idea to send your father to your sister over there? What does your father wish to do? Would he be more comfortable with family and friends at home in India or in USA where he might feel isolated? What type of cancer does he have? Would he require a prolonged treatment or a short swift operation to cure his cancer? All these points are very important to consider before you take any decision. Generally speaking, I do not advise my patients to go abroad for medical treatment, unless the patient himself is very keen to go and financially capable. Moreover, even if a cancer patient takes treatment in USA, later on he is bound to need local Indian doctors and hospitals for the long-term management of his disease.

Q.14: What is Tibetan Medicine? Does it work for cancer?

A: Tibetan Medicine, TM, is a system of herbal medicine developed in Tibet long time ago. This system is similar to Ayurved emphasizing on mind-body connection in disease, life-style changes, dietary changes and lastly herbal formulae for various types of patients and their illnesses. Like Ayurved, TM also describes three humors (dosha), viz. Wind (Vata), Bile (Pitta) and Phlegm (Kapha). Diagnosis is made by history and examination. Pulse diagnosis and urine examination are an integral parts of TM. Different herbal formulae are dispensed to the patients depending upon the diagnosis. These tablets are to be taken three times a day with water. Periodic changes are made in the medicines as per the response of the patient.

There is no simple Yes or No answer to your question whether TM works in cancer. Cancer is a complex disease. TM is aimed at restoration of the internal balance in body enabling it to fight disease. These medicines do not kill cancer cells directly. As a complementary treatment, Tibetan Medicine is worth a trial.

Q.15. My father was operated for tongue cancer and then given radiation and chemotherapy 6 months ago. Now a new gland has appeared in the lower part of neck. Doctors want to give more radiation and possibly more chemotherapy later on. Please let us know if we should follow this advice.

A: Recurrence of tongue cancer and its' spread to lymph nodes in spite of full allopathic treatment is not rare. Depending upon the details of previous radiotherapy, a short second course of radiation can be given; avoiding previously radiated area as far as possible. Whether this will control the cancer remains to be seen. Chemotherapy, which has not worked the first time, can probably be declined since it is bound to produce more toxic side reactions with a very slim chance for tumor control. A lot depends upon the patient's condition and his readiness for further treatments. In any case, you should consider complementary therapy with Ayurvedic medicines to boost up his general condition and improve quality of life.

Q.16. Recently a friend of mine gave me some information about a mushroom product for treatment of cancer. We are thinking of trying it on my mother, who has got a cancer of uterus. Would it help?

A: Mushroom treatment, which originated in Japan, China and Korea, is now becoming popular all over the world. There are many thousand varieties of mushroom; only few have medicinal value. Maitake, Shiitake and Reishi are three important varieties of medicinal mushroom. Originally procured from forests as wild mushrooms, these are now being commercially cultivated in mushroom farms. Mushroom is considered more as a health restoring food supplement rather than a medicine. It does not act specifically against any disease. However, mushrooms are proved to improve cellular function, oxygenation, immunity and detoxification. Indirectly, mushrooms are known to help in many chronic diseases including cancer. In addition to the routine conventional cancer treatment, it might be worth trying mushroom supplements for your mother who has got cancer of uterus.

Q.17: My brother has got a gland size of a lemon in the axilla. Our family doctor insists that we should show my brother to a surgeon for biopsy. We have always taken Ayurvedic treatment for all our family members. Our Ayurvedic consultant says we should not operate. He feels confident that the gland will go away with Ayurvedic treatment. Whom should we follow?

A: We do not know what type of gland your brother has in axilla. It is important to know whether it is due to infection, benign tumor or cancer. The treatment will vary greatly in each case. I would suggest your brother should undergo a biopsy with pathological testing of the gland. Depending upon the report, further treatment can be considered.

Q.18. Can we refuse chemotherapy treatments advised to us by a specialist for the treatment of liver cancer in my father?

A: Accepting or refusing any treatment suggested by the doctors is entirely as per your choice. However, you should choose or refuse any treatment after getting detailed information about possible results of the treatment. A doctor should answer all your questions satisfactorily as far as possible. You may also get more information in this matter from the books, from the experiences of other patients who had such treatments and from other doctors. You have to weigh possible benefits against possible hardships. Chemotherapy is of temporary and marginal benefit in liver cancer. It does not cure liver cancer. Cost-benefit ratio, although considered a bad word in medical field, has to be assessed by the patient.

Q.19: What more can we do to help our mother recover from cancer of breast? She was operated and recently completed a course of chemotherapy. Her general condition has become very weak?

A: I assume that the cancer has been removed and at present she has no residual tumor. I do not know if any chemotherapy or radiotherapy was given to her. These therapies increase free oxidative radicals in body that lead to weakness and toxicity. Your mother would need a lot of supportive care now to recover her strength. Nutritional supplements with natural vitamins and minerals, anti-oxidant supplements, amino acids, essential fatty acids, fresh fruits and vegetables, light & easy to digest diet, Ayurvedic tonics such as Shatavari Kalpa, Badam Pak,

Chyavan Prash etc would help. If she has got poor appetite or any other problems, it is better to consult an Ayurvedic physician. She might need additional herbal and ayurvedic medicine to help her recover faster. You have to keep her under periodic check-ups of your oncology doctors to make sure that the cancer has not recurred.

Q. 20. We hear a lot about Aloe Vera these days? What is that? Does it help in Cancer treatment?

A: Aloe Vera is a thick leafy common green shrub. It grows wildly at many places and can be cultivated for commercial or home use. From the thick leaves, a clear paste like matter is taken out for medicinal use. In Sanskrit it is called Kumari and in Marathi- Koraphad. It is a great liver tonic. It improves liver function, which is essential for normal metabolism in body. It is also used for local applications in ulcers, burns and wounds. It helps digestion and stimulates immunity. The Ayurvedic medicine- Kumari Asav is made from Aloe Vera. Aloe Vera is also available as a dilute juice and as extract in a capsule form. It can be used as a nutritional supplement or herbal supplement for health maintenance. It can indirectly help as a supplementary treatment in cancer because of its' above listed properties.

Q. 21. What is immunity? My father was in good health all his life. My mother died 1 year ago at age 67. My father has now been diagnosed to have cancer of prostate. A friend of mine said that my father does not have immunity that is why he developed cancer. Is it possible?

A: Immunity is a natural disease fighting power in the body. It is a system of special white blood cells and tissue cells that act as police force to detect and destroy any unhealthy activities in body. In health, immune system is very efficient and sensitive to detect any "terrorist" activities in any part of the body, instantly. T-lymphocytes, B-lymphocytes, Natural Killer Cells, Macrophages, Interleukins etc are the components of the immune system. As soon as an "Enemy" is detected, immune cells send signals to other cells for help. In short period of time, a whole police force can gather at the site for the fight. Fight against the enemy is won by capturing the enemy cells and germs, neutralizing the toxins, and ultimately by destroying the offenders. Immunity is of many types and could have many components. A person may be immune to some diseases but may not be immune to some other conditions. Vaccination is one of the methods to stimulate immunity against certain infections like tetanus, measles, small pox, chicken pox, diphtheria, influenza etc.

When a foreign substance is introduced in the body, immune cells react and form what is called anti-body. The initial offender is called antigen, since it initiates the creation of antibody. Antibody attacks the antigen and neutralizes it. Later on the captured and altered antigens are eliminated from the body.

If immune system is deficient, cancer cells somehow evade this weakened immune system and start growing and spreading. Immunity is not a constant force and it is liable to vary from time to time. Good nutrition, exercise, mental happiness, good sleep are known to improve immunity, while lack of these things would reduce the immunity. Mental shocks and painful life events also reduce the immunity.

In the case of your father, who was in good health, the death of your mother might have been a very painful event that affected the immunity and triggered the cancer process. Cancer like cells are all the time wandering in the body, but with efficient immunity, these are detected and destroyed before producing a disease. Depressed immunity, on the other hand, is not able to deal with such criminal cells, which grow unchallenged in to a visible cancer tumor.

You have to understand that a person in good health could still have a weakness only in a part of immunity responsible for cancer. On the other hand, people who get frequent illnesses due to low general immunity may not necessarily get cancer. Low immunity can manifest in a variety of illnesses, cancer being only one disease.

Q. 22. What is colostomy? Doctors are planning a colostomy on my father who has got cancer in rectum. Do we have to do it?

A: Colon is the large intestine that follows after the small intestine. At the lower end, colon becomes rectum through which the stools are discharged from the body. Colostomy means opening colon and bringing one end on the surface of abdomen. When a cancer tumor in the lower part of colon completely blocks the downward passage of the stools, a diversion is made for directing the stools. This is called as colostomy, which is a minor operation that can even be done under local anesthesia. Through a small incision in lower part of abdomen on the left side, a loop of colon is brought to the surface. Then the loop is opened and upper end of the loop is kept open and stitched on the surface of the abdomen. Through this portion, stools can be passed or removed daily by the patient. If this diversion is not done, the patient will develop complete intestinal obstruction due to accumulation of stools in belly. This would be a very serious condition. Colostomy, by providing a diversion, relieves this problem. Colostomy is sometimes temporary, which can be closed later on after removal of the obstructing cancer lower down. If the cancer cannot be removed or if the lower colon has to be totally removed in an operation, then the colostomy becomes permanent, something the patient has to live with all his life. If your father were developing intestinal obstruction, then it would be necessary to do this operation. Please discuss the details with your surgeon.

Q. 23. Does acupuncture help in treatment of cancer?

A: Acupuncture is a part of Traditional Chinese Medicine, TCM. This system describes meridians, which are very subtle invisible channels traversing various parts of the body carrying vital energy to different organs. In Chinese, Chi means vital energy, which is Prana energy. Meridian system can be compared with the internal road system in a cit, which is responsible for proper traffic of goods and persons in all the parts of the city. Energy supplied through the meridians help the normal function of all the internal organs. If a road is blocked, there would be slowdown and traffic congestion. Similarly, if a meridian were not functioning properly, there would be imbalance in the traffic of the energy within the body. If not corrected, this would cause various illnesses. A meridian out of balance can carry either too little or too much energy. Both the situations can lead to various symptoms and diseases. On the surface of human body, the actual path of meridians can be traced at certain points. These specific points are called acupuncture points. Inserting small needles at these points can restore the balance of circulation of Chi or Prana. Blockages in meridians can cause pain in related parts of the body. Acupuncture treatment usually helps to decrease pains. Acupuncture has been shown to relieve other symptoms like nausea, vomiting, fatigue, weakness, cramps, irritability etc. Whether acupuncture on its own can reduce cancer tumor is doubtful. Acupuncture can be used under a trained acupuncturist, as a complementary treatment for symptomatic relief.

Q. 24. My mother always took homeopathic remedies for all her problems. Six months ago she developed a lump in her breast. The lump is increasing under homeopathic treatment, but she is otherwise quite comfortable. Nobody can tell from outside that she is ill. What should we do?

A: Your mother had kept good health, which could be due to many factors; homeopathic medicine could be one of them. Homeopathic remedies at times, by the "law of similars ", are known to cause increase in the tumor size. However, you need not feel guilty about using homeopathy. All the systems have some good and some weak points. It is difficult to say which way the lump will progress. At present, you should consider operation to remove the lump and have it studied by a pathologist. Further treatment can be decided upon final diagnosis of the breast lump. With the help from your family doctor, you should explain various possibilities to your mother and let her take the final decision about her treatments.

Q.25. Is there any cure for cancer in Alternative Medicine?

A: There is no definite guaranteed cure for all the cancers in any system, either in Alternative Medicine or in the Conventional Medicine. A "cure" depends upon the patient, his mental attitudes, upon the efforts the patient would take to help himself, support from cooperative family and finally upon the proper guidance from doctors. At present, integrated approach combining conventional therapies with complementary alternative therapies would be the best course to follow.

Q.26. What can we do to reduce nausea and loss of appetite in my mother, who is under chemotherapy?

A: Nausea and vomiting are common problems experienced by the patients during the course of chemotherapy and radiotherapy treatments. Supplements of large doses of vitamins (especially A, C and E) and minerals should be taken to reduce the toxic free radicals liberated during these cancer treatments. These toxic radicals are partly responsible for many side reactions. Nausea is experienced due to irritability of stomach and intestines. A household remedy consisting of equal parts of shredded ginger, lemon juice and honey taken a teaspoonful at a time before mealtimes usually helps to reduce nausea and vomiting. A homeopathic remedy, Ipecac in 6X, 12 X or 12C taken 15 minutes before mealtime is also found to be helpful to reduce nausea and improve appetite. If these simple remedies do not work, you should use one of the allopathic medicine for nausea / vomiting in consultation with your doctors.

Q. 27. My sister has lost all her hair after chemotherapy? Will the hair grow back?

A: Loss of hair is a common problem during chemotherapy. Some chemotherapy drugs routinely produce hair loss, while certain drugs may spare hair. Please discuss about this with your chemotherapist. After completion of the chemotherapy cycles, hair will usually grow back within 2 to 4 months. Please consider application of a natural / Ayurvedic hair oil containing Brahmi, Awala etc. to the head daily.

Q. 28. My doctors insist that I should eat a lot of high protein food frequently during day. I do not have good appetite. I am recovering from radiation treatments for my prostate cancer. Eating heavy food bothers me. Is it essential that I force food on myself?

A: Unless your digestive power (Agni) is normal, eating a lot of heavy, high protein food would not help. The improper digestion of such foods may even cause other medical problems. First try to improve your appetite and eat food as per your appetite. It is better to eat a little less than to eat too much. Do not force food upon yourself. There are certain Ayurvedic herbs to stimulate your appetite, Agni and digestion. Consult an Ayurvedic physician in this matter.

Q.29. Do you believe in Spiritual Healing? Does it cure cancer?

A: I believe in any method that can help patient heal. Healing is a nature's mystery, which probably depends equally upon innate mental strengths as well as external treatments for a disease. All the methods, conventional or alternative, are based on some assumptions and theories. When it works, that method is hailed as the right one. Obviously, sometimes deliberate frauds are performed by practitioners of various methods for monetary gains. This should be condemned. However, to dismiss any method out of ignorance is not very scientific, either.

Spiritual Healing is based on the principle that every living thing is enveloped in an energy sheath. Invisible to human eye, this subtle body can be called variously as an astral body, vital body, sookshma sharira, linga-deha, aura etc. The health and function of the physical body depend upon health of the subtle body. Most of the diseases start due to disturbances in this sheath. A spiritual healer can either feel or see these abnormalities. A successful spiritual healer can correct the defects and clear up the blocks in subtle sheath, thus helping the person to recover from his illnesses.

A successful spiritual healer can correct the defects and clear up the blocks in subtle sheath, thus helping the person to recover from his illnesses. Dr. Geoffery Morell, a spiritual healer from Washington DC, has visited us in Mumbai several times and given demonstrations of the spiritual healing to our patients. He could correctly locate the disease process in the body by mere passing the hands around the body. His observations would tally with the findings on scans and x-rays, which we did not disclose to him earlier. Even without taking full history of the patient, Dr. Morell could often describe various problems the patient might have had in the past or is having currently.

Spiritual healing is a cleansing process of the subtle body. This is not a permanent cure for any disease. The patient has to work hard to keep his spirit, mind and emotions clean and healthy; otherwise the dirt can accumulate again. It is like house cleaning, which needs to be done periodically. We have noticed significant improvement in various common complaints after the sessions of spiritual healing. In my own case, painful arthritis of my left knee, which did not respond even to steroid injections into the joint 2 years ago, was greatly relieved by a session of spiritual healing from Dr. Morell. Previously unable to walk even for a 100 meters because of pain, I can now walk comfortably even for a couple of kilometers a day. The old bones and old joints are still there, but the pain is gone!

I would not suggest that you should rely on spiritual healing alone for cure of cancer, which needs a multi-pronged attack. Spiritual healing could help you in a complementary way to remove any blocks and negativities in your subtle body. The success depends upon ability of the healer as well as your faith and receptivity.

Q. 30. I am 50 years old man and work as a manager of a manufacturing company in Mumbai. I wish to go for cancer check-up. What will they do?

A: various hospitals and doctors offer routine medical check-ups to health conscious people, who may be in apparently good health. Many companies even pay for health check-ups for their employees. The Indian Cancer Society and some other private hospitals also offer Cancer check-ups. You should initially have a general medical check-up, which would include some basic blood tests, cardiogram and chest x-ray. Consultant physicians of each hospital will then examine you. You might be asked to undergo more tests if needed, depending upon your initial assessment.

In cancer check-up, you are given basic blood tests, X-rays and a detailed examination by cancer doctors to rule out any obvious tumor or ulcer process. Depending upon the findings, further tests might be ordered to clarify any doubts. If your cancer check-up comes normal, that means you do not have any obvious cancer clinically in the common cancer areas of the body. If you are above 50 years of age, you may consider having a medical check-up and cancer check-up. However, cancer is a slow growing process, which takes years to manifest as a visible tumor. One normal cancer check-up will not guarantee that you would be always free of cancer. You would need periodic check-ups, say once every 3 to 5 years. The best thing to prevent cancer, however, is to embark upon a healthy life-style, good nutrition with natural foods that fight cancer, regular exercise, positive mental attitude and above all a feeling of happiness about you, whatever you are.

Q. 32. There is history of cancer in my family. I am worried about cancer. Can I do anything to prevent cancer?

A: Cancer cells have abnormal genes. One could be born with susceptible genes, which are prone to develop cancer later on. This way, there is some increased risk of cancer if one has got many blood relatives with cancer. However, the good news is that most of the times, by avoiding exposure to cancer triggering factors called carcinogens, one can reduce the risk of cancer in spite of having abnormal genes. Healthy life-styles, proper nutrition with cancer fighting foods, regular exercise, good hobbies, positive mental attitude would go further to minimize the cancer risk. Remember, most of the times, your own bad habits have caused increased risk for cancer. Replacing improper habits with good ones will certainly help you prevent cancer. Such precaution might even keep your "faulty genes" from developing cancer. The details of causes of cancer and preventive steps are discussed at length in earlier chapters of this book.

Q.33. I hear a lot about mind-body medicine for cancer. What is it?

A: Mind-Body medicine is a recently coined term but it has been practiced, knowingly or unknowingly, by many complementary alternative medical sciences. Mind is what makes the physical body act. Mind cannot be seen but we know it is somewhere there. Diseases affect both the mind and body. Directing treatment only at pathological disease process, as is usually done by allopathic medicine, might not produce satisfactory results in chronic diseases, which might have deep roots in the emotional/ mental level. Mind- Body medicine advocates attention to both these inseparable components.

Yoga, meditation, visual imagery, biofeedback, reiki, spiritual healing, therapeutic touch etc are some of the techniques used in Mind-Body Medicine. The idea is to strengthen your own mind to improve your immunity, to remove negative feelings and instill healthy emotions to improve your health. Of course, you would also need actual physical therapies for the physical part of your disease process.

Q.34. Does magnet therapy work in cancer?

A: I have not seen magnet therapy alone curing cancer. Application of magnets in a particular way to body parts is supposed to align and energize iron containing organic molecules, especially hemoglobin in the blood. The practitioners of magnet therapies claim various benefits. I personally do not have any experience giving magnet therapy. Therefore I am not in a position to comment, either positively or negatively, about magnet therapy. It is probably harmless and possibly beneficial, if done under guidance of a practitioner having expertise in this area.

Q.35. Why do patients get side reactions of radiation treatments? Is it true that radiation itself is a cause of cancer?

A: Radiation is a beam of ionizing radiation energy that causes a variety of strong biochemical and physical changes in cells. It liberates toxic radicals, which in turn interfere with various normal cell functions. Cancer cell, due to rapid growth, are destroyed by the radiation energy more than the normal cells. After radiation, normal cells recover faster while cancer cells recover slowly, if at all. The toxic radicals as well as the products of cell destruction circulate in the blood and reach different organs. With high doses of radiation, the organs in direct beam of radiation develop reactions like burning, irritability, ulceration and even loss of function. Apart from these local reactions, there are general reactions like loss of appetite, weakness, fatigue, nausea, vomiting, heat etc. These reactions start appearing during the second week of radiation course and continue till end of radiation treatments, after which reactions subside within 4 to 6 weeks. However, some residual changes like hardening of skin, thickening of the part under radiation, reduced blood circulation etc are left for a long period. Some patients have to live with these changes for the rest of the life.

Radiation can cause genetic mutation, which alter the genes. Some of these mutations, if not repaired by the body, could cause cancer after a period of 7 to 10 years. This happens in less than 5% of the patient undergoing radiation. However, this is a significant risk a patient has to accept for the treatment of his cancer with radiation.

Q. 36. What kind of side effects can happen due to chemotherapy drugs? Is there any way to prevent side effects?

A: Chemotherapy is administration of strong drugs, either by mouth or by injections, to destroy cancer cells. These drugs also destroy normal cells to a lesser extent. Chemotherapy drugs circulate through the whole body and therefore the side reactions are also more wide spread than those in radiotherapy. Loss of appetite, weakness, burning sensation, loss of hair, nausea, vomiting, diarrhea, sores in mouth, pile like symptoms etc are common side reactions of chemotherapy. Certain drugs produce specific toxicity to heart, lungs, bones, nerves, kidneys etc. That is why chemotherapy is given only by expert oncologist with frequent blood tests to avoid extreme reactions. Like radiation, chemotherapy drugs also can cause mutation in genes, which can possibly cause a cancer later on after a gap of some years.

Good nutrition, liberal supplements of vitamins and minerals, large amounts of liquids etc would reduce incidence of reactions. There are some specific allopathic medicines that your doctor could prescribe to reduce some of these reactions. There are effective medicines in Ayurved and Homeopathy to decrease the severity of side reactions. You should take these medicines with consulting appropriate practitioners.

Q: 37. It is difficult for us to look after our father who is suffering from terminal cancer. Is there any hospital or nursing home we can admit him in?

A: For a terminal cancer patient, when there is no other treatment possible, few special centers called hospices are available. These are routine in the developed nations. In Maharashtra, two such centers are doing wonderful job of making the life less painful and less miserable in the last days of the illness. Shanti Avedana Ashram in Bandra (Mumbai) and Cipla Cancer Aid Foundation, at Warje (Pune). There may be some more centers in other parts of India but I do not have details at present. These centers would help cancer patients and their relatives about the terminal care of cancer patients.

Q.38. My father is very angry in nature. He has developed a stomach cancer. He blames us that we are not taking good care of him. It is very difficult to cope up with him. Any advice?

A: It is very difficult task for relatives to take care of cancer patients, especially the angry ones. These are trying times for all. Patient should look at the cancer as an opportunity to discover new meaning to the life and resolve old conflicts. This is easier said than done. Relatives should learn to be more sympathetic, kind and helpful to the patient at such times. There is no use arguing with your father in this matter at this stage. You cannot change him. With patience and kindness, try to show that you all love him and are ready to do everything possible. Perhaps he is trying to take out his frustration and disappointment with life with the angry spells. His angry nature might have contributed to the development of cancer in the stomach, the organ closely affected by anger and insecurity.

Q.39. My 70 years old mother has developed cancer of throat. She is a very religious, pious and kind personality. She will go out of her way to help anyone in need. We wonder why God is so unjust to punish good persons with diseases like cancer.

A: God's ways are strange. Human mind cannot logically explain many incidences in the world. We do get angry with God when we see a small baby suffering or when an innocent person a victim. In your mother's case, there might be some suppressed emotional conflict or self-neglect in nutritional matters (so common of Indian housewife) that might have triggered the cancer. It could be the genes that underwent spontaneous mutations and caused the cancer. It could be some medicines she took earlier in her life or the injuries, mental and physical, she might have suffered earlier. It is hard to explain. Finally, we can always point our fingers to the FATE!

Q. 40. Why small babies, who never had any bad habits or cancer causing substances like tobacco etc, develop cancer? Is this not a paradox of Divine Justice?

A: In childhood cancer, there is more likely-hood of being born with abnormal cancer prone genes, which express to develop cancer in young age. The genetic mutations could be due to exposure to toxins in the womb of the mother during pregnancy. It could be due to some inherited genetic weakness. It could be even explained as Karma from past lives, if you believe in re-births. It is painful to see an innocent child in pain due to cancer. It is hard to understand divine justice. You can only have faith to be at peace.

Q. 41. What is Wagholi Project of Cancer Research?

A: Guided by Poojya Sardeshmukh Maharaj from Pune, his son Vaidya Sadanand Sardeshmukh and myself developed a protocol for cancer treatment at the Ayurved Hospital and Research Center at Wagholi, about 20 km east of Pune. This project has been running since 1994 and has enrolled more than 1200 cancer patients over the past 7 years. We have seen that Ayurvedic medicines can greatly help to reduce side reactions of cancer treatment, reduce pain and improve general condition of cancer patients. Ayurvredic treatment, which alone may not be able to cure cancer, is used as an addition to conventional cancer treatments as surgery, radiotherapy and chemotherapy. Detailed information of this project is given in earlier chapter "Ayurved For Cancer" in this book.

42. Is Bhallatak (Bilawa-Bibwa) good for cancer treatment?

A: Dr. B. G. Wad, a senior physician from Mumbai, did extensive research on use of Bhallatak, an herbal nut used frequently in Ayurved. Dr. Wad found it useful in treatment of certain types of cancers. A product called Anacarcin was developed by Bombay Pharmaceutical Company. This product is no longer available. Recently Ethichem Laboratory in Ahmedabad has come up with Anacarnex, a product made out of Bhallatak. Bhallatak has several properties and can be tried as a complementary treatment.

Q. 43. Can I try Heerak Bhasm (diamond bhasm) for my cancer?

Yes, you could try this under supervision of an expert ayurvedic physician experienced in the use of Heerak Bhasma. Ayurvedic texts have given many properties for Heerak Bhasma and it is possible that this might have some benefit as a complementary treatment. However, I would not rely only upon Heerak Bhasma, if I had a cancer.

Q.44. Should I continue heavy exercise, which I was doing before I was diagnosed of having cancer of bones?

A: If the cancer has affected your bones, you should refrain from any heavy exercise that may put on strain on your bones. Heavy exercise may produce fractures at the site of bone cancer, a very problematic and difficult situation to handle.

Q.45. I am a 15-year-old boy. I fell down from cycle and injured my right knee one year ago. For last few months I am slowly developing a hard painful swelling around the lower part of my right knee. Could this be bone cancer? What should I do?

A: Many times, old injuries leave weakness in the part involved in such injuries. Although apparently the injury heals, the area is at a risk of developing disease later on with minimal provocation or disturbances of dosha. Some chronic diseases are known to occur later on in athletes and boxers who suffer repeated injuries during the professional career. Falling off from the bike is a common incidence in teenagers. Not all the swellings are due to cancer, but it should be investigated. It would be a good idea to take an X-ray of the knees to rule out any serious problem. If there are any doubts, MRI scans can provide much better information than an X-ray film. You should consult an experienced orthopedic surgeon for examination and detailed advice.

Q.46. My 8 years old son suffered a head injury 3 years ago. He had a concussion at that time and was in hospital

for 2 days for observation. There was no fracture seen on X rays. Last month he developed continuous headache. A CT scan shows a tumor in the left side of brain. Doctors have advised operation. Can tumors happen due to old injury?

A: Tumors can result from old injuries. Not every head injury results in brain tumor but in a significant number of brain tumors, there is history of old head injury. Brain tumors are commonly benign, which can be cured after surgery. A small number is due to malignant tumor, for which additional treatments might be needed. If your doctors advise operation, you should consider the same for your son.

Q. 47. Is Pancha-karma Ayurvedic treatment good to treat Caner ?

A: Pancha-Karma is a part of Ayurvedic treatment that is undertaken to extricate disturbed dosha out of body. It is a sort of body purification method that removes the toxic waste products and dosha, which are at root of a chronic disease process. Pancha-Karma are five fold purification methods, which should be done under proper supervision of an experienced ayurvedic physician.

Q. 48. Should the doctors treating cancer worry about the expenditure of the costly cancer therapies?

A: Doctors should be concerned about the possible expenditure of costly therapies. Cost of the current medical treatments and investigations is beyond an average hard-working honest Indian salaried person. Health insurance, to reimburse the hospital bills, has not yet become common in India. Even in advanced countries like USA, a significant number of unemployed people are not able afford a personal health insurance.

A patient should openly ask and the doctor should freely discuss the cost benefit ratio of the long-term expensive medical care in a disease like cancer. Expensive treatments may not necessarily cure cancer. If there is a good chance of controlling the cancer in a patient, you should accept all the treatments you can afford. In advance stage of cancer, there is no use of subjecting the patient to costly treatments, which might prolong the life but by a few months only, unless patients and relatives are keen to go to such extent. At this stage, quality of life, peace and symptomatic pain relief is more important than trial of new radiotherapy or chemotherapy techniques. Relatives wish to do everything possible for the old parents to have all possible treatments regardless of the cost. Do not forget what a parent wishes. Do not force your wishes on the parents or elderly relatives. Respect the wishes of a terminal cancer patient who wants to avoid all those pains, side reactions, tubes and needles all over the body at the end. Sometimes expensive treatments are undertaken out of pressure from the relatives and friends. There might a "guilt complex" associated with saying NO to expensive treatments of doubtful benefits. The matter of the expenses, although a secondary issue, should be given careful thought when the outcome of such treatments is not certain.

Q. 49: What is your opinion on Euthanasia (mercy killing)

A: Some medical and social activists in different parts of the world advocate euthanasia by allowing doctors to give large doses of sedatives to terminate life, if terminal patient is in severe pain and discomfort and if he so wishes to die. This is a very controversial topic. Although few European nations have legalized such procedure, laws of most nations do not permit active "mercy killing". There are various ethical, legal and technical issues involved in euthanasia, which can be misused.

I am against the concept of active euthanasia. However, passive euthanasia, withdrawing all the emergency life support systems, when a patient in misery expresses his consent is acceptable. Withdrawal of all the tubes, needles and respirator support from a patient in emergency ward might hasten the end. This might be preferable, rather than artificially prolonging life for a short period, from the viewpoint of the patient and relatives. Discussions about such issues should be openly done between relatives and the doctors. A patient can sign in advance a "No Resuscitation Request" to indicate his wish under such circumstances.

Chapter 15

TERMINAL CARE

There comes a time, for all of us, to face death. Death is the other side of the coin we call life. Life and death of physical body follows in cycles. Although death is a bad word, one cannot avoid it. One can think and prepare about a decent, peaceful and noble death. Death is nod defeat, it is only and end of the current chapter in unfinished book of own eternal life. It is only the physical body that dies. If there were no death, imagine what kind of the world there would have been. There would be stagnation, boredom and lack of new fascinating future possibilities. After certain number of years, physical body deteriorates, like any other machine. With good maintenance (self care) and good brand (good genes), you might hope to use this machine longer but not forever.

In the second chapter of Bhagawad Geeta, the Hindu Scripture, Lord Krishna says, " As a man discards old torn up clothes and puts on new ones, similarly discarding the old diseased physical body, the soul takes up a new body (to continue on his path of karma)". Although the thought of death is terrifying, it is a transitory experience one has to go through, again and again, till one reaches the GOAL of eternal peace, power and happiness. There are other couplets stating the laws of Karma to explain all the possible incidences in this universe. Having scientific bent of mind, which demands a proof for every theory, many people might not accept such doctrines. Detailed discussion on Karma theory is out of the scope of this book.

As stated earlier, death is not failure. Failure is not to take the challenge of disease to do all possible efforts to fight the enemy. These trying times teach a lot to the main actor as well as to close helpers and the spectators in this eternal drama of life and death.

The main concerns in the care of the terminal cancer patients are as follows:

1. How far one should go in trying different treatments?
2. Should expenditure be a consideration?
3. Should a patient be removed to a hospital when apparently there is no specific treatment?
4. Is home care possible for the terminally ill?

In a terminal patient, different treatments have probably been already tried and found not useful. That is why the case has become terminal. At this stage, patient's peace and comfort are most important. Any heroic treatments, which will be physically painful to patient, could be declined. Safe, gentler natural treatments could be considered to give symptomatic relief and to improve the quality of life as far as possible. Liberal doses of pain killer medicines such as morphine and other analgesics could be used if needed for severe pain.

Expenditure for providing peace and comfort to the patient is worthwhile. Sometimes, refusal to agree for an expensive treatment produces guilt complex in relatives of the patient. If one can afford, and if such treatment is not going to be worse than the disease, it could be undertaken as a trial. Spending more money does not necessarily produce better results. In terminal care, comfort of the patient is the most important thing to worry about. The merits for prolonging life, which might be already burdensome, by a few more days, weeks or months by intensive treatments, should be discussed amongst the relatives and due respect should be given to the patient's own wishes.

In the terminal care, focus should shift from anti-cancer treatments to mind-body medicine, music therapy, relaxation, reading, introspection about own life and resolutions of conflicts if any. Cheerful friends could make a great difference. Patients might have different inclinations, different interests and different hobbies. Not each patient might like to spend last days in meditation, japa and coming closer to the spiritual truths. Relatives have to cater for each patient as per his inclinations and provide maximum cheer, humor and peace.

Hospices are specially developed medical facilities to provide care for the terminally ill. Here the emphasis is not on treatment of the cancer but on making the remaining short span of life more comfortable and peaceful. Trained doctors, assisted by a dedicated staff of nurses and social workers, run such facilities, where a patient can be admitted for short period of time. Attention is given to adequate pain relief and providing a friendly noble and peaceful atmosphere. Dr. L. J. D'Souza, a well-known cancer surgeon from Tata Memorial Hospital, started Shanti Avedana Ashram, a terminal care center in Bandra, Mumbai. Dr. Anuradha Sowani, a prominent medical oncologist from Pune, started a terminal care center at Warje-Pune, sponsored by Cipla Pharmaceuticals from Mumbai.

These centers are doing a great job to make the life easier for terminally ill cancer patients and for their relatives .For more information about these centers, you may phone:

1. Shanti Avedana Ashram, Mount Mary Road, Bandra, Mumbai, Phone: 022- 642-7464 / or 642- 1889
2. Cipla Cancer Center, Warje- Pune, Phone (020) 612-7837, or 612-8336

For symptomatic relief, hospitalization for a short period may be needed. Emergency surgical procedures like tracheostomy, colostomy, gastrostomy, aspiration of fluids from chest or abdomen, urinary catheterization etc are best done in a nearby hospital. It is often observed that in terminal stages, prolonged hospitalization against the wishes of a patient brings the death closer.

Sometimes, the relatives are afraid or unable to take care of the patient at home. In such a case, admission to a nearby nursing home or hospital may be necessary. However, at terminal stage, hospitalization may be a mentally traumatic event for some patients, who would rather pass the last days at home in familiar surrounding. It is a complex issue but if the relatives are able to look after the patient at home, that is usually the best solution. For this, one would need support from a mature sympathetic and friendly family doctor and nurses in the neighborhood.

One can consider hiring nursing aids and Aaya to look after the patient at home. Home care is the best solution in terminal stages if the patient so wishes and if the relatives are able to provide this.

Death should be dignified, peaceful and respectful to the Inner Person.

Chapter 16

COMPREHENSIVE CANCER CARE CENTERS

PROPOSAL FOR INTEGRATIVE CARE

WHY?

War Against Cancer needs a multilevel attack for success.

There are hundreds of published papers confirming the benefits of integrating Complementary Alternative Medicine (CAM) with conventional cancer therapies. Time has come for us to seriously integrate such evidence based complementary alternative medical methods in our hospitals and medical colleges to serve our patients better. Such programs based in medical colleges would also provide a great opportunity to our medical students to learn about CAM and to serve their patients better when they start their careers. Leading hospitals and cancer centers should think of establishing such units.

AIMS & OBJECTIVES:

1. To combine evidence based complementary medical methods in the treatment.
2. To educate cancer patients and their relatives about various treatment options.
3. To promote clinical research trials to explore the role of CAM in cancer.
4. To educate medical community about various options in cancer treatment.

5. To provide to the patients other services such as psychological support, group support, home care, terminal care, pain clinics, accommodation and transport etc.

WHAT?

CAM methods most commonly employed in cancer are:
1. Mind Body methods: Meditation, relaxation response, biofeedback, guided imagery, visualization, reiki, therapeutic touch are few examples.
2. Support Group Therapy: Exchange of information, personal experiences and guidance by professional health care providers has shown to benefit cancer patients and their relatives.
3. Physical methods such as Yoga, Exercise, Movement Therapies, Physical Therapies, and Massage have demonstrated useful supplementary role
4. Nutrition has been proved to be a key factor in causation as well as prevention of cancer. Use of antioxidants and specific supplements is very important.
5. Ayurveda
6. Acupuncture
7. Homeopathy

FEASIBILITY

Considered impossible only a few years ago, the idea to create integrated facilities to provide cancer patients different complementary alternatives is now taking hold all over the world. Departments of Integrated Medicines have been started in various renowned medical schools in USA and Europe. Pioneering work for such integration to provide better care to cancer patients has already started at the following world- renowned American hospitals.

1. Patient Network Services, at the M.D. Anderson Cancer Center in Texas

2. Center for Integrated Therapies, at Dana Farber Cancer Center in Boston
3. Complete Care Program, at Fox Chase Cancer Center
4. Integrated Medicine Service, at Memorial Sloan Kettering Hospital, New York

There are many more similar integrative initiatives in USA and Europe. India, a country with rich heritage of Ayurved, Homeopathy, Yoga and many other Mind-Body Medical Methods, is in a unique position to develop Integrated Medical Centers attached to various prominent medical institutions. These units could offer choices of safe, effective, natural and affordable medical care to countless millions. Indian mind is (usually) open and tolerant to different paths. If open-minded Indian doctors from various disciplines come together in cooperative fashion, this task would be done easily.

HOW?

A general plan for establishment of Comprehensive Cancer Center (CCC) is available. This would be modified as per the needs, available facilities and nature of cancer workload peculiar to each hospital or medical center. A committee of experts may be formed to finalize the development of Comprehensive Cancer Center at each center. The committee may consider how best to combine various CAM methods in various current cancer treatment protocols. The committee may consider how to promote the aims and objectives of CCC as stated above.

A special unit called Comprehensive Cancer Center is to be established. Existing medical and paramedical facilities are to be fully utilized. New personnel can be recruited for specific work assignments.

The CCC may invite help from and various specialists dealing with cancer

A. Oncologists: Surgeons, Radiation Oncologists and Medical Oncologists

B. Cancer research scientists from disciplines like pharmacology, pathology, biochemistry, clinical nutrition etc.

C. CAM practitioners of Ayurveda, Homeopathy, Acupuncture and others,

D. Social Workers,

E. Yoga & Exercise teacher, Massage therapist etc.

It is difficult task in the beginning. However, as the time goes, many prominent medical centers in India would be able to develop such integrated centers for the great benefit of health care of Indians. .

Chapter 17

CONCLUSION

Each patient must fight the War Against Cancer, enthusiastically and fearlessly, with support from the family, friends and above all competent medical practitioners. Although a dreaded disease, cancer process can be reversed by proper attention to the core, the fundamentals and the therapies described in earlier chapters. The subject is vast and at times confusing. Faulty nutrition and bad life styles can trigger cancer. Good news is that correcting nutrition and life styles can reverse the process of cancer.

Cancer is getting commoner because of several factors, external as well as internal. Pollution, toxic wastes in environment, chemicals in food air and water, Tobacco, atmospheric radiations, are some of the external factors. The internal factors are mental stress, emotional conflicts, blocks due to negative attitudes, disappointments, frustrations and deranged internal metabolism of the body that forces the body to store the toxins in various organs. These external as well as internal factors interfere with normal immunity and can even lead to genetic mutations, which are at the basis of malignant transformation of cells. Human body has many natural defense and repair mechanisms. With persistent onslaught of the offending factors, there comes a flash point starting the process of cancer disease.

Many novel methods to detect cancer cells at a very early stage are available. When cancer tumor, even a small one, is seen on medical examination or X-rays it already a collection of millions of cancer cells! Blood tests based on detection of cancer antigens would be better than X-rays and scans for early detection of cancer.

Cancer affects Mind- Body apparatus and therefore has to be fought at both these levels. The core of cancer treatment lies in Mind/ Body medicine to resolve any emotional conflicts and to strengthen the mind to fight the battle. Foundation of cancer treatment rests on improvement in life styles, nutrition, exercise, relaxation and detoxification techniques to remove the accumulated toxins in the body. It is a sort of basic groundwork one needs to do before starting any definitive anti-cancer treatments. In a hurry to start a treatment such as surgery, radiation or chemotherapy, attention to the core and foundation is often neglected. To get better results and long term control of cancer bordering on "cure", addressing the core and foundation is essential.

Various Complementary Alternative Medical methods practiced by different doctors and scientists are mentioned separately in the chapter on Treatment Options. The proponents of each method have advocated most of these approaches. Confirmation of consistent benefits from most of these methods will need further scientific proof by more clinical research trials.

Two specific CAM methods, Ayurved and Homeopathy, have been dealt with more details in separate chapters. Psychological trauma and negativities is an important factor in causation of cancer that needs adequate attention for a good outcome. Examples of some actual patients with unusual psychological disturbances and remedial actions are given in the chapter on " Psychology of Cancer".

The chapter on "Frequently Asked Questions" provides brief answers to various common questions from cancer patients and their relatives. The chapter on "Terminal Care" provides few useful tips to deal with the difficult situation at the end. Suggestions for establishments for Comprehensive Cancer Centers in various prominent cancer centers are given in one of the last chapters.

I hope that this work will provide a lot of information on cancer and all its aspects. It would help the patient and the relatives to deal with cancer with better understanding, less confusion and less terror. The information in the book should also help any reader to understand about prevention of cancer and other chronic diseases. This work is for your information only and should not be taken as a suggestion of a specific treatment for a specific cancer patient. You will need to consult your doctors for specific path to follow. There are no guarantees of success implied in this book.

Let us end this presentation with the famous Prayer from Veda:

Let Everyone Here Be Happy and Healthy
Let Everyone Be Free From Disease
Let Everyone See Noble Things
Let No One Have Sorrows

Aum Shanti, Shanti, Shanti: PEACE

APPENDIX: 1

CHECK LIST FOR ACTION

Following general instructions are written for attending the core and fundamentals of health maintenance. Following these directions is expected to improve general health, immunity and feeling of well being. Acting on these instruction would reduce risk of cancer for an average person. This would also help reverse the cancer process in a patient.

Attitude:
Cultivate positive attitude. Count your blessings rather than brooding over problems. Be concerned about your health but not worried about it. Affirm daily that you love yourself as you are. Respect and love others. Do not blame others and do not find faults with others for your predicaments. Accept responsibility for whatever happens in your life. You are the creator of your own destiny. Be confidant that you are going to overcome any and all the problems with your own will, determination and efforts.

Belief:
Analyze your belief systems. Belief and faith are what make life progressive and worthwhile. If you believe in God, pray for direction and help for your battle. If you do not believe in God, ponder over what you believe in. All the knowledge and logic is supported by the basic belief in your own existence. Try to find who you really are. Meditation is the tool to explore the inner universe. Dry logic and arguments do not lead you to the goal of your life. Look at your illness as an opportunity to find new meaning, new directions in your life.

Goal:
Fix up a material goal that you would really like to achieve in a time bound manner. Abstract goals like " I want to be happy", " I want to reach Nirvana", " I want to help people", "I want to get detached" etc are not adequate to give your mind the incentive to be positively

occupied. Focused cheerful mind can be a great tool for regaining health. A goal could be any specific material achievement, which might add to your self-esteem.

Relaxation:
Develop some hobbies like music, debating, reading, photography, travel, sightseeing, dancing, games etc that could make your life more pleasurable. Seek company of good friends and develop social circles. Attend performances of drama, dances, music and other cultural arts to uplift your mind.

Nutrition:
Nutrition is not only about eating good foods. Digestion, assimilation and elimination are the three processes, which should be efficient for proper nutrition. Appetite must be good to digest the foods properly. If appetite is poor, any good food will be of little use. Overloading the system with food could create metabolic toxins to hamper your health further. Following are some ways to improve the appetite, digestion and overall nutrition. .

1. Do not overeat; always stop eating just before the stomach is very full. You should develop the habit of listening to your stomach rather than following your tongue.
2. Do not eat until you are hungry. Follow a schedule for regular mealtimes.
3. Periodic fasting can stimulate Agni and appetite. You may skip a meal once in a while to tune up the stomach fire- jatharangni.
4. Take a teaspoonful of mixture of fresh shredded ginger, lemon juice and pure honey before mealtimes.
5. Develop regular habits for exercise, work, relaxation and sleep schedules.
6. Avoid or reduce non-vegetarian food intake.
7. Eat plenty of seasonal vegetables and fruits. Prefer organically grown farm products if available. Organically grown food products avoid use of chemical fertilizers, pesticides and

insecticides that can contaminate food chains and enter your body. Eventually, these can accumulate in tissues.

8. For proper colonic cleansing, take mild herbal laxatives periodically. Even if you are not constipated, herbal laxatives can help your body detoxify. However, do not overuse laxatives, which can produce dehydration and weakness. Consult an Ayurvedic physician for proper guidance. Triphala, Haritaki, Sukha-sarak Churna are some of the herbal laxatives recommended in Ayurved.

9. Drink large quantities of plain pure water, 2 to 3 liters daily. This can help disposal of waste products from body.

Nutrition For Mind:

Good thoughts, healthy emotions and company of good people are important for mental health. We are very careful to provide good food for the body. We should be even more careful to provide good food for the mind. Try to analyze your own mind and strive to become a better person. Mental negativity is one of the fundamental causes of many chronic illnesses. A person who feels internally happy rarely develops chronic health problems. Develop sincere love and respect for others so that you could get same thing in return. Try to help others whenever you can. Sincerely serving others without pride is a sure way to subdue personal ego.

Breathing:

Learn and practice the techniques of deep abdominal breathing. This can improve the oxygen supply of the cells. Cancer does not grow in well-oxygenated tissues. Learn other techniques of Pranayama if you are interested. Focused breathing can greatly help concentration and calming of the mind.

Exercise:

Exercise is very important for circulation, immunity, function, strength, vigor and overall health. Find your own level of exercise with which you would be comfortable. At the least, develop habit of daily brisk walking for about 30 minutes.

Immunity:

Attention to all the above points will improve your immunity that is the disease fighting power. Make healthy changes to your life-style. You are the architect of your own health and happiness.

Finally, remember, the body has to eventually die. Death is Not a Failure. Not accepting challenge of life is the real failure. Death is not the end-all. Life is for learning, experiencing, achieving and progressing. Live life fully, cheerfully.

APPENDIX 2

DIET TO FIGHT CANCER

Once a rare disease, cancer is now widespread, affecting large numbers in all the nations. The rise in cancer has paralleled the rise in factory farming and use of processed foods containing vegetable oils, artificial preservatives and food additives. The best approach to cancer is prevention. Bad foods can increase the risk of the cancer. Good foods can reduce the risk of cancer and even reverse the cancer process.

Traditional diets containing natural fresh farm products produced organically by nontoxic methods are rich in factors that protect against cancer. Consumption of generous quantities of seasonal fresh vegetables, fruits and whole grain foods would provide protection against cancer. When possible, prefer organically grown foods to commercially grown agricultural products that use pesticides, insecticides, antibiotics, hormones and chemical fertilizers.

It is probably unnecessary to focus the attention on individual micronutrients. A well-balanced natural diet containing seasonally available fresh fruits, vegetables, whole grains, dairy products, proteins and fats would help reduce cancer risk and promote general health. The diet should be light and easy to digest. In some cases, high doses of vitamins and nutritional supplements might be necessary for a short period of time until a proper diet can be assimilated naturally. These supplements might be especially helpful during the courses of radiotherapy, chemotherapy and convalescence. Please consult a physician for appropriate supplements and vitamins for you.

You should include following health promoting items in your daily diet. This list not exclusive and there might be many more items helpful for good health.

1. A small quantity (10 to 20 gm) of dry fruits: Almonds, cashews, pistachio, walnuts, raisins, dates, figs, black raisins etc

2. A small quantity of good quality fats, ghee, flaxseeds (linseeds),

3. Daily intake of one or two fruits (between 50 to 100 gm): apples, oranges, pineapple, papaya, guava and any other seasonal fruits

4. Vegetables: fresh green leafy vegetables, cabbage, sweat potatoes, carrots, tomatoes, beet, radish, pumpkin, cauliflower etc

5. Sprouted beans (moong, mutki), Wheatgrass,

6. Fresh buttermilk promotes digestion, provides nutrients and acidophilus (friendly bacteria) for improvement in intestinal health. Some fermented foods also provide friendly bacteria.

7. If appetite and digestion are poor, take 1 teaspoon of freshly shredded ginger, honey and lemon juice in equal parts for a few days before mealtime and repeat when necessary.

8. Use spices like turmeric, cumin, coriander (dhania), cinnamon, cloves etc in cooking to make food tasty and to improve digestion.

It is advisable to avoid foods made from white refined flour, white sugar, bakery products made out of white flour, vanaspati ghee, saturated fats, pop drinks, canned foods, foods containing artificial flavors and colors and foods containing chemical preservatives. Avoid deep fried foods. All these items are detrimental to the health. These items are hard to digest and could lead to toxic wastes in the body.

Table indicating micronutrients in various foods and their actions:

Micronutrient	Found In	Action
Beta Carotene	Carrots, yellow and green vegetables, sweet potatoes, Spinach and leafy green vegetables	Protects against all cancers, especially Cancers of cervix uterus and lung
Vitamin B-6	Bananas, leafy green vegetables, apples, Sweet potatoes,	Maintain immunity, health of mucus membranes, barrier to pollution, protect against infection, Help detoxification
Vitamin C	Citrus fruits, lemons, oranges, Apples, cantaloupes, green peppers,	Maintenance of healthy immune function, Protects against cancers,
Vitamin E	Dark green vegetables, eggs, wheat germ, unrefined vegetable oils, nuts, wheat grass,	Powerful antioxidant, reduces free radical damage, acts against damage done by ozone and smog
Selenium	Fruits and vegetables,	A trace element that helps production of Glutathione, an enzyme essential for detoxification, fights cancer
Folic Acid	Beet roots, cabbage, leafy vegetables, eggs, dairy products, citrus fruits, fish	Synthesis of DNA and RNA, constituent of the genes and chromosomes of nucleus of cells
Calcium	Dark green vegetables, nuts, seeds, grains, milk products, fish	Formation of healthy bones and teeth, blood clotting, cellular metabolism, protects against colon cancer
Iodine	Seafood, sea vegetables as kelp, spirulina, algae,	Growth and repair of all tissues, thyroid function, energy metabolism, protects against breast cancer

Magnesium	Nuts, fish, green vegetables, whole grains, brown rice,	Protects against cancer, maintains blood pH, Synthesis of RNA and DNA, nerve function,
Zinc	Whole grains, seafood, sunflower seeds, soybeans, onions	Protects against prostate cancer, needed for RNA and DNA synthesis, immune function,
Allicin & Alliin	Garlic (fresh or aged) and garlic oil,	Protects against cancers of stomach, esophagus, colon and lung, Helps immune enhancement
Omega-3 Fatty acids	Flaxseeds, Linseeds, nuts, dry fruits, fish, vegetable oils,	Essential for formation and function of all the cells and tissues, Protect against breast cancer, arthritis, inflammations,
Fiber	Whole grains, fiber rich foods, vegetables, legumes, beans	Helps detoxification of colon, protects against cancer of colon,
Vitamin A	Butter, Eggs, Dairy products, fish, nuts,	

APPENDIX- 3

WEBSITES FOR ONLINE HELP FOR CANCER

Following are few important websites that provide a wealth of information and further links to other sites. You need to be familiar with the use of Internet to access these sites on your computer. The sites give information about views of modern medicine (allopathic conventional medicine) and also of complementary and alternative medicine about cancer problem and treatment. This should be used to obtain more information about cancer and other diseases. The author does not recommend use of any specific treatments for your health problems. You should consult your physician for validity of any particular line of therapy you wish to explore in a specific situation.

1. National Center for Complementary and Alternative Medicine, USA
   www.nccam.nih.gov/
A part of National Institutes of Health of US Government devoted to research about complementary and alternative medicine in various health conditions. Provides wealth of information about all the aspects of alternative medicine. Archives list thousands of research publications in this field.

2. National Cancer Institute, USA
   www.nci.nih.gov/
Another important agency in National Institutes of Health devoted to cancer. A wealth of information about various types of cancer, current recommendations, ongoing research, information about various medicines etc is available.

3. M. D. Anderson Cancer Center, University of Texas, Houston, TX 77030, Phone 1-800-392-1611

www.mdanderson.org/departments/CIMER
Complementary & Integrative Medicine Educational Resources for cancer.

4. Center for Mind Body Medicine, Washington, DC, USA
www.cmbm.org/
Information available on alternative and integrative medicine with emphasis on mind-body medicine. Proceedings of annually held Comprehensive Cancer Care Conferences can be viewed on this website.

5. Cancer Control Society, Los Angeles, CA, USA
www.cancercontrolsociety.org/
Devoted to find Alternative Medical solutions for Cancer. Lists various centers and practitioners in this field.

6. Dr. Burton Goldberg, a researcher in alternative medicine and editor of several books.
www.alternativemedicine.com/
For information on Complementary and Alternative Medicine on Cancer and many other diseases.

6. God Help Me! : Cancer Survivors Book
www.godhelpme.com/
Information about cancer survivors and guidance on various matters in cancer treatment.

7. American Cancer Society, USA
www.cancer.org/
World-renowned cancer society to help cancer patients on various fronts.

8. Indian Cancer Society, L.R.Tata Medical Center, M. Karve Road, Mumbai 400021,
Phone: 022-202-9941, Fax: 022-287-2745
www.indiancancersociety.org/

For information about cancer in India and various activities to help cancer patients in India.

9. Cancer Patients Aid Association, Mumbai, India
      www.cpaaindia.org/
Actively engaged in helping cancer patients for guidance, counseling, help with transport and medicines etc.

10. Jeevan Jyot Cancer Relief & Care Trust, Mumbai, India
      www.jeevanjyot.org/
Charitable trust helping cancer patients in various matters.

11. Ayurved Hospital & Research Center, Wagholi, Pune, India, Phone: Mumbai: (022)4130866
      www.ayurved-for-cancer.org/
A branch of Bharatiya Sanskriti Darshan Trust established in 1954 to promote ancient Indian Arts and Sciences. Research and treatment with Ayurved is an integral activity of this trust. Cancer Research Project with Ayurvedic Treatments started since 1994. Website has information on their projects on Ayurved for cancer and many other diseases. Phone: Pune 020-67346000, Mumbai: 022-4130866

There are many more institutions and organizations doing very important work in this field. It is not possible to mention them all. Interested persons may do search on Internet with appropriate WORD.

APPENDIX-4
Books & References For Further Reading

I have referred to following books and publications for some of the information given in this book. This list is only partial. These books further list thousands of research publications on various areas of cancer.

1. Alternative Medicine Definitive Guide to CANCER,
Burton Goldberg, W. John Diamond, M.D. and W. Lee Cowden, M.D., Future Medicine Publishing, Inc., Tiburon, CA, Published in 1997

2. OPTIONS: The Alternative Cancer Therapy Book,
Richard Walters, Avery Publishing Group Inc., Garden City Park, New York, Published in 1993

3. MANFESTO FOR A NEW MEDICINE,
James S. Gordon, M.D. Perseus Books, Reading, MA, Published in 1996

4. LOVE, MEDICINE AND MIRACLES
Bernie Siegel, M.D. Arrow Publication, Published in 1988

5. HEAL YOUR BODY, Louise L. Hay, Hay House, Inc., Carsbald, CA, Published in 1988

www.ingramcontent.com/pod-product-compliance
Lightning Source LLC
Chambersburg PA
CBHW070002300526
45794CB00001B/158